PRAISE FOR
YOGA OFF THE MAT

"*Yoga Off the Mat* is the book I wish I'd had when I first started yoga. While there are many books on yoga philosophy and the sutras, this one stands out for weaving the esoteric with the practical. It's both a guide to practicing yoga and to living well. Too often yoga is confined to the mat, but this book invites us to step off and make every action a practice. That reminder feels more essential than ever in today's world."

—GABRIELLE HARRIS, author of *The Inspired Yoga Teacher, The Language of Yin,* and *Lessons in Meditation*

"Yoga isn't just postures you do on your mat. It's a complete philosophy, a set of ideas and guidelines to take you to union with the Divine—the true meaning of yoga. This book covers all the basics and is a must-have for any yoga practitioner. . . . If you need to bone up on yoga philosophy or want a spiritual teacher in written form, this book is for you."

—ANODEA JUDITH, author of *Wheels of Life, Chakra Yoga,* and *Eastern Body, Western Mind*

"An important contribution to making the heart of yoga practical and accessible. *Yoga Off the Mat* touches on a wide range of yoga philosophy in a format that's phenomenal for beginners and more seasoned yogis ready to take their practice to the next level. The concept is brilliant—apply these ancient teachings to your busy life. This is how transformation happens, and this book can be your companion."

—ANN SWANSON, MS, author of the best-selling *Science of Yoga* and *Meditation for the Real World*

"Given the liberatory nature of yoga and the current sociopolitical landscape, now more than ever it is essential that yoga practitioners consider how to engage their practice more deeply and fully. One way to do this is to immerse oneself in deeper study beyond the physical asanas of the yogic path, and to combine the knowledge learned through this immersion with action in the world. Sage and Alexandra have taken what can feel like very dense material based on philosophical frameworks and ancient contexts and made it applicable and accessible. Their teachings in *Yoga Off the Mat* inspire yoga practitioners to expand their understanding of yoga, therefore living the path more fully."

—MICHELLE C. JOHNSON, author of *Skill in Action* and *Illuminating Our True Nature*

YOGA OFF
THE MAT

ALSO BY SAGE ROUNTREE AND ALEXANDRA DESIATO

Teaching Yoga Beyond the Poses

Teaching Yoga Beyond the Poses, Volume 2

Lifelong Yoga

ALSO BY SAGE ROUNTREE

The Art of Yoga Sequencing

The Athlete's Guide to Recovery

The Professional Yoga Teacher's Handbook

The Runner's Guide to Yoga

Everyday Yoga

Racing Wisely

The Athlete's Pocket Guide to Yoga

The Athlete's Guide to Yoga

ALSO BY ALEXANDRA DESIATO

Whole Mama Yoga, coauthored with Lauren Sacks

YOGA OFF THE MAT

A PRACTICAL GUIDE TO THE WISDOM OF YOGA

FIND BALANCE, MEANING, AND LIBERATION IN YOUR DAILY LIFE

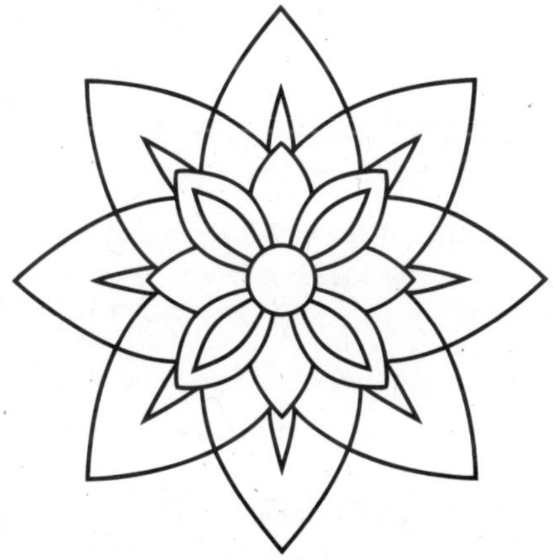

SAGE ROUNTREE & ALEXANDRA DESIATO

ILLUSTRATED BY LASHA MUTUAL

North Atlantic Books
Huichin, unceded Ohlone land
Berkeley, California

North Atlantic Books
Huichin, unceded Ohlone land
2526 Martin Luther King Jr Way
Berkeley, CA 94704 USA
www.northatlanticbooks.com

Cover photo © S.Zahan via Adobe Stock
Cover design by Jasmine Hromjak
Book design by Happenstance Type-O-Rama

Printed in Canada

Yoga Off the Mat: A Practical Guide to the Wisdom of Yoga—Find Balance, Meaning, and Liberation in Your Daily Life is sponsored and published by North Atlantic Books, an educational nonprofit that collaborates with partners to develop cross-cultural perspectives; nurture holistic views of art, science, the humanities, and healing; and seed personal and global transformation by publishing work on the relationship of body, spirit, and nature.

North Atlantic Books's publications are distributed to the US trade and internationally by Penguin Random House Publisher Services. For further information, visit our website at www.northatlanticbooks.com.

The authorized representative in the EU for product safety and compliance is Eucomply OÜ, Pärnu mnt 139b-14, 11317 Tallinn, Estonia, hello@eucompliance partner.com, +33757690241.

Library of Congress Cataloging-in-Publication Data
Names: Rountree, Sage, 1972– author | DeSiato, Alexandra, 1979– author |
    Mutual, Lasha illustrator
Title: Yoga off the mat : a practical guide to the wisdom of yoga—find
    balance, meaning, and liberation in your daily life / Sage Rountree and
    Alexandra DeSiato ; illustrated by Lasha Mutual.
Description: Berkeley, California : North Atlantic Books, [2026] | Includes
    bibliographical references and index. | Summary: "How to bring yogic
    wisdom and philosophy into everyday life for deeper meaning, balance,
    and joy"— Provided by publisher.
Identifiers: LCCN 2025054952 (print) | LCCN 2025054953 (ebook) | ISBN
    9798889843603 trade paperback | ISBN 9798889843610 ebook
Subjects: LCSH: Yoga | Self-care, Health
Classification: LCC B132.Y6 R678 2026 (print) | LCC B132.Y6 (ebook)
LC record available at https://lccn.loc.gov/2025054952
LC ebook record available at https://lccn.loc.gov/2025054953

1 2 3 4 5 6 7 8 9 FRIESENS 31 30 29 28 27 26

To the seekers and the knowers,
who are one and the same.

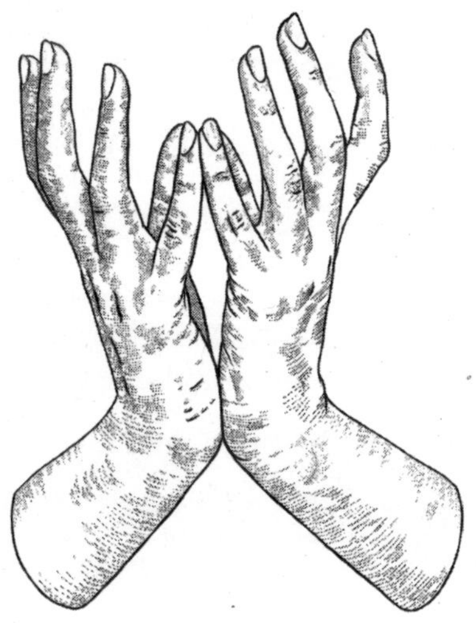

CONTENTS

PREFACE

Millions of people turn to yoga for flexibility, fitness, and stress relief. But what if the most transformative part of yoga isn't the poses at all? The true power of yoga is found in its underlying philosophy—wisdom that can help us navigate our biggest challenges, find freedom in daily life, and create deep, lasting balance. Yoga gives us a framework for life and offers a sense of meaning, clarity, and connection. But too often, modern yoga focuses only on the poses, leaving out the wisdom that makes it transformational.

This book bridges that gap.

We are yoga teachers and former academics with over fifty years' combined experience sharing philosophy to help our students make sense of their existence—whether it's in a college English classroom or on a yoga mat. While students may come to yoga for a workout or a stretch, they come *back* to yoga because it offers them a feeling of meaning and wholeness. This book is here to enhance that connection.

Yoga Off the Mat will help you understand how yoga philosophy is not only relevant to your practice but can be the key to finding freedom, meaning, and balance in life. Indeed, for the modern yoga practitioner, practicing the poses without a foundational understanding of the philosophy behind the practice is tantamount to kneeling in prayer to an unknown god. So much of modern yoga is focused on the physical practice, but that focus is a limited, and misguided, interpretation of an ancient practice. The shapes you are making with your bodies aren't the entire story, and the path to liberation doesn't have to include sun salutations—unless you want it to! As teachers, we know students of yoga are hungry to put their practice into context and to find deeper meaning on and off the mat.

Yoga Off the Mat offers accessible yoga philosophy that's immediately applicable to the daily, modern life of a yoga practitioner. We hope you will finish this book with a practical understanding of yoga's core philosophies and how to integrate them seamlessly into your life—whether that's using the mindfulness techniques of *pratayahara* and *dhyana* for stress, reframing challenges with yogic wisdom like *pratipaksha bhavana,* or deepening your personal practice beyond the movement of *asana,* the physical poses. The advice in the book will help you navigate your workplace, family life, and spiritual life—our hope is that it offers you a sort of sacred life raft in the challenging and ambiguous times we live in. We aim to offer thoughtful, elegant historical wisdom packaged in a way that is readable, relevant, and absorbable for anyone who has hungered to understand more deeply why yoga is so moving, freeing, and enlightening.

We wanted to create this book together because the philosophical and spiritual lessons of yoga are foundational to *our* daily lives and worldviews. We walk through the world with yoga as our lens; in our best moments, that means we operate from a place of nonharming, compassion, and acceptance. (And in our worst moments, we at least know what we're aiming to get back to as our *modus operandi!*) Even if you have a different, existing faith practice or religion, there is space for yoga to be part of your divine bedrock. The versatility of yoga as a spiritual framework is that it can coexist with other faiths. And it's not dogmatic: You don't have to adhere to every single element, suggestion, or ethical precept in the many ancient texts that intertwine through the thousands of years of history of yoga. Instead, you get to mindfully and analytically consider their major themes and determine what could help you live a kinder, better, more present life in the modern world. That's not cherry-picking; it's recognizing that yoga is an active, living, unfolding system, and as we deepen our knowledge of the foundational philosophy of yoga, we can allow our key takeaways to reflect that evolution.

Our earlier books *Teaching Yoga Beyond the Poses* (2017) and its second volume (2025) are designed for yoga *teachers,* offering them practical ways to weave yoga philosophy into their teaching through themes and messages that resonate with students. This book, on the other hand, speaks directly to yoga *practitioners*, helping you integrate yoga philosophy—which can often be intimidating—and your personal practice.

Yoga Off the Mat provides tools for individual self-reflection and application. We hope that you take what works for you. While many yoga books focus on either yoga poses or dense philosophy, this book offers a middle path. We hope to provide you with insights and practical takeaways that will resonate with you and be applicable in your daily life and across a broad range of settings: intra- and interpersonally, at home, at work, and out in the world. We end each chapter with practical actions to take your yoga beyond the poses and into your daily life. These short, doable actions—reflections, small habit shifts, or journaling prompts—help you bridge the gap between philosophy and practice. Our goal is for you to not just understand these ideas but put them to use in your life.

YOGA OFF THE MAT

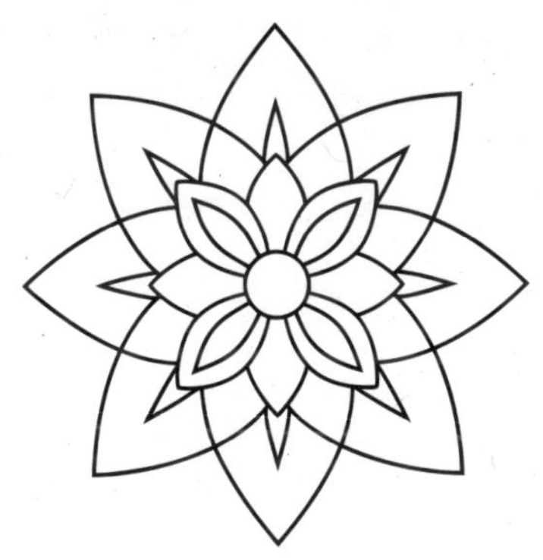

INTRODUCTION

Before you dive into this book, please note that while we are both scholars, we are not extensively or solely scholars of yoga philosophy. Our degrees in English literature reflect our desire to understand the range of human experience and to investigate how to live life well—often through storytelling and wordplay. In writing this book, our desire is to extrapolate the ideas that resonate deeply with us as decades-long yoga practitioners and teachers, rather than to provide a text that covers the breadth and depth of yoga thought. Scholarly texts that encompass all yoga philosophical thought *do* exist, and they are written by and for other scholars. We're writing for everyday yogis in what we hope is a colloquial, inviting, warm voice.

Let's start with a little history: You can't make sense of yoga philosophy without being able to envision the historical timeline of that philosophy. Knowing that these spiritual practices are truly ancient gives them even more weight and power—especially when you begin to recognize that they still have significant meaning for our daily lives. The goal of this introduction, then, is to guide you through the vast history of yoga, so you can understand where these ideas come from and, from that, how they still apply to you millennia later. In *The Yoga Tradition*, scholar Georg Feuerstein writes,

> *India's chronology is notoriously conjectural until we come to the nineteenth century. The Hindu historiographers have seldom been concerned with recording actual dates and tended to mingle historical fact with mythology, symbolism, and ideology.*[1]

Trying to create a coherent sense of yoga history is challenging both because of what Feuerstein notes and because yoga has been around for a long time. Yoga is between three thousand and five thousand years old, and the important books of yoga—including the Vedas, Upanishads, Yoga Sutras, and Bhagavad Gita, which you've probably heard of, if not yet encountered—are only a few of the myriad of ancient texts (and various versions and translations of those texts) that explain yoga practice and theory.

Another reason it's hard to truly date where yoga began is that it didn't start in recorded form; much of early yoga consisted of philosophical ideas passed down orally from guru to student, sometimes in a secretive environment. We call the early era of yoga the "pre-Vedic" era, because it predates a group of books called the *Vedas*. In this pre-Vedic era, we have no textual evidence of yoga. What we have, instead, is some imagery of deities and meditation. Some scholars argue that this suggests a starting point for yoga, which continues into the eras that follow centuries afterward.[2]

This brings us to the Vedas—an important group of yogic texts. There are four Vedas. But to say that there are four Vedas is sort of misleading. Imagine, for a moment, your favorite cookbook. You probably use it extensively. In this beloved cookbook, each recipe is probably not entirely unique. Each recipe has likely been adapted, culturally influenced, changed by historical trends, and altered due to ingredient availability in various regions. In fact, *you've* probably changed the recipes as you've tried them, substituting in vegetables you prefer or spices you have on hand. This is a great way to imagine the Vedas: Each one is a cookbook, and the recipes have been added over time. These recipes were initially passed down orally, then changed, updated, rewritten, and reenvisioned depending on the chef, reader, writer, environment, and available ingredients. So, while yoga scholars identify four Vedas—the *Rig Veda, Samar Veda, Yajur Veda,* and *Atharva Veda*—each Veda is really a collection of "recipes" about rituals, healing, hymns, chants, mythology, and protection that have been updated and altered over time.[3] And in the Vedas, we see the seeds of what grows into yoga. (Indeed, the first use of the word *yuj,* the root word of *yoga,* meaning "to yoke," is in the *Rig Veda.*)

Yoga philosophy sits alongside five other classical Indian philosophical systems, and it's influenced by its philosophical cousins. This is familiar territory. Have you heard the phrase "everything's a remix"? This is a perfect example of that. In the same way that American democracy is based on ancient Roman and Greek governance systems and draws from Enlightenment philosophical ideas, yoga draws from the prevailing philosophical and spiritual practices in the region of the world where it evolved. Hindu iconography often pervades yoga spaces, and Hindu mythology is woven through the stories, chants, and mantras common in yoga. You've probably noticed that Buddhist ideas and yogic ideas are similar and, in some cases, the same. These spiritual practices and faiths were coming into existence at the same time as yoga did—evolving alongside it, influencing it, and broadening its spiritual scope. How, then, did yoga grow from these classical roots into our modern, physical, Western, women-dominated practice?[4]

The last portion of the Vedas is the Upanishads, which contain philosophical wisdom. Sometimes the philosophical sentiments of the Upanishadic period are referred to as *Advaita Vedanta*, literally "end of the Vedas." We might envision the Vedas as a tree and the Upanishads as the fruit that tree bears: The Upanishads are the distillation of the ritual ideas in the Vedas into a form that is full of nourishment and sweetness for the seeker. The Upanishads are the mystical complement to the Vedas. In the Upanishads, contemplation and meditation are offered as a path to *moksha*, or liberation—an idea we still see alive in our yoga practices today.

Another key point of the Upanishads might be summed up like this: You are not in the universe; the universe is in you. The Upanishads argue that your innermost essence is not separate from the vastness of reality. In this way, the Upanishads present a nondualist view of spirituality. (In fact, the veil of separateness is *maya*, an illusion.) Sometimes in modern-day yoga, we talk about *prana* (life force) being both a vast sea (all of existence) and encased in a jar in that sea (an individual, in the confines of their body, immersed in existence). You can see how this latter idea arises from the former.

You may have heard the phrase "classical yoga" before. Sometimes this refers to all yoga that existed before modern yoga, but it generally points to a specific time in yoga history: the period of the Yoga Sutras. If you've encountered no other yogic text, it's likely that you've at least heard of ideas from this one. The Yoga Sutras is probably the most-referenced ancient yogic text in the modern day, and the reason for that is twofold: It is both brief and relatively accessible. The author of the Yoga Sutras, the sage Patanjali (or perhaps just as likely, a group of writers over time who then attributed their work to one sage), had a goal of distilling the most valuable points from the yogic texts that came before into a briefer manual which could be used as a life guide. Because of its relative succinctness, it's also accessible for modern readers who might get lost in the ritual details of the Vedas or elaborate contemplative mysticism of the Upanishads.

The ideas of the Yoga Sutras are ones you've likely heard before, such as the eight limbs of yoga, which point to a "path" of yoga practices we can incorporate for greater bliss and freedom, or the yamas and niyamas, which give us a code of ethics for both how we should treat others and how we should treat ourselves. Each *sutra* (thread) is detailed enough to provide an intricate and rich philosophical meal to enjoy, but it is also brief enough that the reader can adjust and season the meal (interpret its wisdom) to fit their life and circumstances. In many ways, the brevity of the sutras is what keeps them highly relevant today: Each short thread of thought is open to wide interpretation. In fact, when you seek out the actual text of the Yoga Sutras in the present day, you'll find that there are many different interpretations of it. Publications of the sutras generally include a blurb following each sutra, offering commentary by the editor of that edition. A sutra-by-sutra comparison in different books can reveal radically different interpretations of the same short lines!

One of the things that's so fascinating to us about yoga history is how philosophical thinking shifted after the Yoga Sutras, which broadened how yoga approached the concepts of freedom and liberation. Classical yoga and the Yoga Sutras generally emphasize renunciation as an important aspect of the journey toward freedom. Sometimes in our modern readings of the Yoga Sutras, we soften this aspect, but it's a recurring theme of the text. Consider, for instance, that in the Yoga Sutras, three of the eight limbs of yoga are concerned with turning inward, concentrating, and meditating. Consider also that both *saucha*—cleanliness—and *brahmacharya*—chastity—are important ethical guideposts in the Yoga Sutras. All of these point to self-denial and abnegation as a path to deliverance.

The rise of tantra yoga came a few hundred years after the Yoga Sutras. If you read the word *tantra* and immediately connected it to the physical body (or sex!), you're not exactly wrong. The tantric yogis and their texts, like the *Yoga Spandikarika* or the *Vijnana Bhairava Tantra*, moved away from the idea of renunciation as the key to freedom. Instead, they believed that incorporating all aspects of being human was not just possible in a spiritual life but *necessary* for it.

The tantrics rallied around ideas that had drifted through earlier yoga philosophy in the Upanishads and brought them to life with renewed spirit. Where the Yoga Sutras saw the physical and spiritual as separate, tantra yoga saw embodiment as the key to divinity. This chapter of yoga philosophy sees the physical body not as an obstacle that needs to be overcome or purified but as a vehicle for liberation. In this, we can see the seeds of our modern asana practice. If you've ever wondered why yoga began as a largely philosophical, meditative practice and evolved into a physical one, tantra yoga helped pave the way for that shift.

Spirituality was nondual in tantric understanding, and that nondualist view of divinity persists in modern yoga. Consider the common teaching that divinity is inside you already; that's nondualist. Another important idea from tantra that we see in yoga today is the concept of Shiva and Shakti. You may have heard this simplified as meaning "masculine" and "feminine" energies, but it's more encompassing than that. Shiva represents the force of the universe that is always observing and always waiting. Shiva is potential, watching from the dark. In contrast, Shakti is the spark of movement and creation. Shakti dances her way over, lights everything up, and coaxes potential into something material. Together they play, explore, create, and dance together, unfurling the cosmos. This dance is called *lila*: It's the divine having fun, relishing in the ways it can create. Perhaps a key point, too, is that this act of creation does not have any specific goal or aim at a particular result. Tantric philosophy tells us that the universe is playing just to play— and our existence is a result of that. For tantric yogis, the goal of yoga is to immediately wake up to the truth of divinity in all of existence.

Tantra gave rise to hatha yoga, which stripped away some of the rituals that accompanied tantric practices and once again simplified things. If tantra's goal was immediate enlightenment and connection with the divine, hatha's goal was liberation by way of harnessing prana in breathwork, meditation, and other practices. Hatha yoga also brought about the democratization of yoga: Prior to this period of yoga, learning about yoga was restricted to ascetics and renunciates. Through hatha yoga, these practices became practices of householders and, later, women. In the medieval *Hatha Yoga Pradipika*, women are even acknowledged as holders of pranic energy through their sexuality.[5] The idea of the energetic or subtle body—models like the koshas, movements of prana, and the chakras—arose from tantric ideas, but this concept was made more accessible through hatha yoga texts and physical practices. The texts that arose in hatha were often manuals of practice that offered detailed suggestions about pranayama (working with the breath) and asana (working with the body).

Hatha is foundational to our modern, posture-focused yoga, which arrived in the late 1800s and early 1900s. To understand how modern yogic culture evolved, you have to know a little about colonialism in India. Our physical yogic culture is the result of revived and reimagined yoga, born from anti-colonialism, Indian national pride, gymnastics, and other forms of movement.[6] Modern yoga founders you've probably heard of like T. K. V. Krishnamacharya, B. K. S. Iyengar, Indra Devi, and Pattabhi Jois brought yoga into the mainstream, first in India and then into other parts of the world, including the West.

As with so many other elements of technology and life, the pace of development and change in yoga has increased exponentially since its introduction to the West in the 1800s. While a yoga studio was still a rarity in an American city in the 1970s, now you can find yoga studios most everywhere. Many of them are franchises with distinct brand elements such as a particular sequence, room temperature, class title system, or other standardized approach. Many of them, like Sage's studio, are small community-focused operations run by teachers who are dedicated to bringing opportunities for connection to their students. Yoga studios offer a foundational place for movement, community, stillness, and communion with spirituality. And, of course, a lot of downward-facing dogs. With the ubiquitousness of yoga came another big shift: Yoga today is practiced and taught largely by and to women.

Our current yoga culture, now led by women, is rethinking the stringent alignment that was such an important aspect of yoga just twenty years ago. There's a richer understanding that human bodies are diverse, and the goal of the physical practice is no longer to make postures uniform across this variety of bodies. Instead, yoga has come to serve as a respite, as self-care, and as an opportunity to rest and unwind. But the spiritual roots of yoga persist in our modern practice: You don't come to yoga with the same mindset or expectations you bring to any other movement practice. In addition to moving your body in a meaningful way, you also come to yoga to feel something deeper or to know yourself better. You come to yoga for *lila*, to play in your body, to be the universe witnessing itself. This is what makes yoga so deeply meaningful. It's probably what had you picking up this book; you recognize there is great power in a yoga practice that has little to do with the exact shapes you make with your body.

Despite these various philosophical shifts, the accelerated pace of adaptation, and the proliferation of new styles, yoga ultimately remains the same: It's a system with very deep, very old roots that seeks to lead practitioners to better awareness and freedom. Whether that's done on a fancy mat in a hot room with black lights, in a town park, on a living-room floor, or in a South Asian ashram, the goal is union (*yoga*) and liberation (*kaivalya*). Yoga philosophy continues to help you move toward this sense of meaning, so that you can rest in your true nature, whole and divine.

PART I

THE YOGA SUTRAS AND A SIMPLIFIED SYSTEM OF YOGA

As we saw in the introduction, the Yoga Sutras are just one small part of the yoga tradition, yet they carry a lot of weight when we think about yoga philosophy. The sutras are a chain of aphorisms that act as a shorthand guide to the practice of yoga. Most of the text needs exposition by a teacher or guide—it's not a page-turner self-help book that you can pick up, understand, and immediately implement. While some of it is clear—even practical—most of it will require several passes over consecutive years, during which time your perspective as a reader will continue to shift. Some of it is just plain out-there: In its later books, the sutras turn to an investigation of the mystical powers, called *siddhis*, that yogis can develop. Let's look at some of the ideas from the sutras you may have already encountered in your yoga classes and consider how you might apply them outside the context of your physical practice.

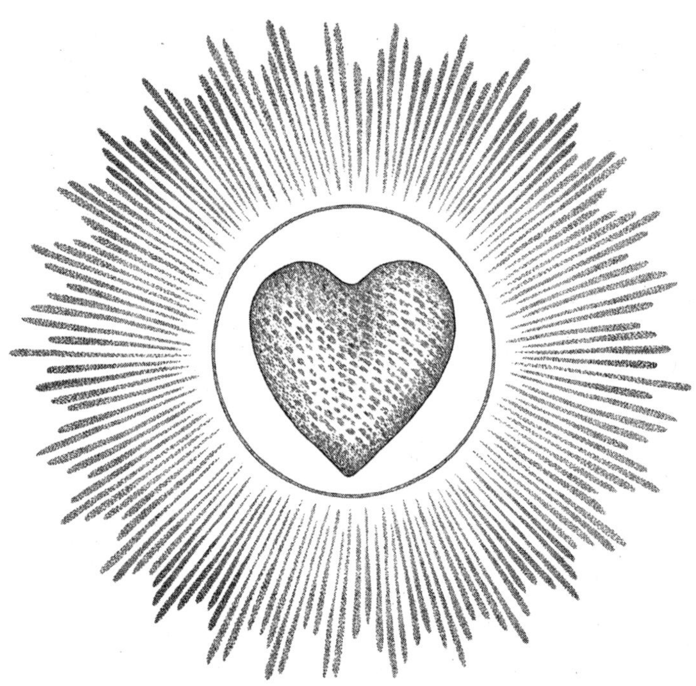

1

AND NOW:
THE STUDY OF YOGA

The first words of the Yoga Sutras are *Atha yoganusasanam: Now, the study of yoga begins.* The study of yoga is *always* about the now, the present. We are in the modern world, and the study of ancient yoga is still relevant, still applicable—you know this to be true, or you wouldn't be reading this book.

What a powerful opening word, *now*. It is a demand for presence as the starting point of the entire practice. *Now* is an attention-getter. Before the streaming era of television, we were accustomed to hearing an announcement of the upcoming program just before it started: *"AND NOW* . . . the HBO original series . . . *Ballers."* Though this may seem like a quaint relic, for many of us, the sound of the TV set turning on and the familiar announcer's voice calling out "and now . . ." was a Pavlov's bell, prompting us to get out of the kitchen, grab the popcorn, and sit down for *The Sopranos,* or *Sex and the City,* or whatever your favorite show was.

The sutras open with this same call: the word *atha,* which means "and now." Your ears are meant to prick up at this word: Here comes what you've been waiting for. Scholars concur that *atha* is a rhetorical phrase akin to saying, "Therefore, given the entire argument I have made to this point. . . ."

The "now" that begins the Yoga Sutras is our first reminder that the entire goal of the practice is to be in the now, to be present to the moment. This is an idea that both of us (as yoga teachers) theme into our classes constantly. That's because it's always relevant; we all need the constant reminder to "be here now," as Ram Dass famously put it. (Or, to put it in pop-cultural terms, we can look to the words of Kung Fu Panda: "Yesterday's history, tomorrow's a mystery. Today's a gift. That's why they call it the present.")

Your mind is an excellent time traveler, and left without the yoke of "now," it will revisit the past, making changes and revisions to your memories, or dart ahead to contemplate the future, making assumptions or projecting anxieties. *Atha* harkens it back to what's happening in the immediate moment.

ACTIONS

Be here now. Sit, stand, or recline quietly for a moment and turn your attention to what is happening now. Notice how quickly your mind wants to move backward or forward, away from the present moment. When it does (which usually takes no time at all), gently direct your attention back to *now*. An anchor for that could be your breath; the points of contact between your body and the floor, your seat, or your bed; a sound you hear; or the quality of light that you see, whether your eyes are open or closed.

The more you hone your ability to redirect your attention to the present, to the now, the more you are learning to bring your full presence and awareness to every situation. If you never make it any deeper into this book, or if you went to read the Yoga Sutras and never made it past the first word, that would still be enough. The more you are in the here and now, the more fully you move toward freedom and liberation.

Begin again. As you begin reading this book, you're in one stage of your self-knowledge and growth. Next month, next year, or next decade, you'll be in another, and you will find this book lands differently with you. Things that felt murky on your first pass might seem blatantly obvious on your next read, or things that feel weighty and inspiring on this read may ultimately feel irrelevant or not applicable to your life the next time you pick up this book.

Great! Because every time you come back to the start, back to yourself, you're practicing yoga. *And now, the study of yoga begins.*

2

QUIET THE MIND

Sutra 2 says, *Yogas chitta vritti nirodhah*. In Sanskrit, *chitta* is the entirety of the mind, including memory, ego, and intellect. *Vritti* means something like fluctuations or movements. And *nirodhah* implies stopping or ceasing. So, when we translate this from Sanskrit to English, we can see this sutra as a definition of yoga: *Yoga is quieting the mind to see yourself.*

The goal of yoga is to still your mind so your true self can be realized, rather than being overshadowed by constant mental activity. (You already know this; isn't this why you came to yoga in the first place?) Indeed, one of the most important gifts yoga offers us is a chance to stop: stop the planning, stop the doing, stop the scrolling on your phone. The practice, whether asana, pranayama, or meditation, is an opportunity to observe yourself existing. (Just observe—not label, change, or even wonder.) The work is not doing, but undoing.

You can see how this second sutra relates to the "now" of the previous chapter: You simply cannot be fully present, fully in the now, if your mind is loud. The most important lesson of yoga is to teach us how to be here, now, with things as they are. With the phrase *yogas chitta vritti nirodhah*, we move from a definition of yoga to the central practice of yoga. It's not just that practicing yoga quiets your mind; rather, the *quieting* is the practice you have to master to truly do yoga. While this is ancient wisdom, we might argue it's a harder practice to master today. Now we are all an arm's reach away from devices that can endlessly and fully distract us. Collectively, we're probably struggling to be present more than ever before. But that's the reason we practice *quieting* through yoga.

Once we begin to recognize the mind's habitual fluctuation and diversion away from what is happening in the current moment, we can start to subdue that chatter, the *chitta vritti*, of awareness or consciousness, the *chit*. (Some iconoclastic teachers like to say this sutra encourages us to get our *chit* together.) When we accept the truth that our consciousness has become accustomed to jumping from item to item, and that in so doing turns us away from our true nature, we can reduce the swing of the pendulum of our attention. We can begin to let our consciousness center around its true still point: the Self, right here, right now, exactly as you are. When we see this Self, we drop our misguided attention to anything that is not the Self.

ACTIONS

Listen to your thoughts. To quiet the mind, you might start, ironically, by thinking. Begin by asking yourself, *Why am I being pulled away from this moment by my swirling thoughts?* This question allows you to see if there's actually something that requires your action or immediate response. Often, quickly writing down distracting thoughts can help you let them go. You'll also have a record of them on hand to come back to once you have finished practicing presence.

For instance, maybe your response to this question is "I'm thinking about the groceries I need to get for tonight's dinner." If that's the case, perhaps you can pause to write a grocery list, knowing that once you do, you can let go of that particular mind-focus. But be discerning; it's easy to create an endless list of to-do tasks from your mind's darting thoughts.

Don't listen to your thoughts. Again, ask yourself, *Why am I being pulled away from this moment by my swirling thoughts?* This time, what we hope you will notice is that usually there is no *real* reason. Most of the time, the things that feel pressing can wait; the concern that feels so urgent is probably manufactured by your ego; the bit of your past you're ruminating on is unimportant (and cannot be changed anyway). When you ask yourself why you're everywhere but *here and now*, you might notice that your swirling thoughts are ones you *can* let go of, at least for the moment.

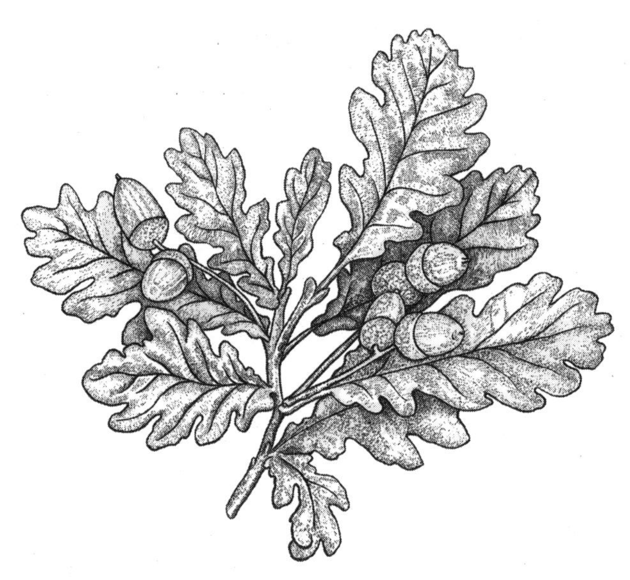

3

A DELICATE BALANCE

Yoga is the careful balance of dispassion (*vairagya*) and dedication (*abhyasa*). It's the balance of practice and detachment, of caring enough and not caring too much. It's the balance of effort and ease. This looks a little different for all of us, but you can probably think of some examples of this in your own life.

While it can be challenging to find the line between nonattachment and continual effort, it's a necessary exercise for you to practice. You have to know that balance for yourself. If you detach too much, you lose the will to continue. If you work too hard, you get too attached to the outcome. Anyone who's ever experienced the many "false starts" of online dating in the modern world has played with this balance: You lean in, express interest, and put yourself out there, but you also do your best to manage expectations and try not to get attached too early. (This can be especially challenging when your mind gets pulled to daydreams of weddings and rocking chairs on porches with your fascinating new prospective partner!)

Trying to balance an appropriate amount of effort and attachment may seem like a frustrating double bind. Think of the "Cool Girl" stereotype: We're expected to put effort into our appearance but act as if beauty comes naturally. We're expected to achieve success but not to let the effort behind it show. But while the imagined Cool Girl persona is one of smoke and mirrors, balancing *vairagya* and *abhyasa* requires you to truly show up as your best self and dedicate yourself to whatever is in front of you, without expecting *anything* in return. If you read that and felt instant discomfort, consider that you may have been raised in a very results-oriented culture, where emphasis was often on the result, not the experience that came through the journey. Consider, too, that focusing on what's to come, rather than what is occurring at the moment, is the very antithesis of being here now—and we've already learned that *now* is the heart of yoga.

ACTIONS

Find the balance, literally. In your asana practice, you're used to quite literally working the line between effort and ease to hold your balance poses. If you approach a challenging balance pose while wanting it desperately, you'll try too hard, and the pose becomes locked down, rigid, and unsustainable. If you are dispassionate to the point of being uninterested, you'll apply too little effort, and you fall right out of the pose. Notice how this plays out the next time you visit tree pose or crow pose.

Find the balance, metaphorically. Look for other areas in your life where you can find a need for balance. It turns up everywhere, once you begin to seek it. Romantic partnerships? Don't smother and cling—but don't go cold. Parenting? Be faithful to the task of loving, guiding, and providing for your children, but also know that they must learn lessons for themselves and make mistakes along the way. Cooking? Try a new recipe with zeal and gusto, but sweetly accept if your family members don't like it. The dance of dispassion and dedication shows up constantly throughout our lives. Practice the moves and you'll become a good dancer.

4

WHERE IS MY MIND?

In chapter 2, we talked about one definition of yoga: quieting the mind. Sometimes we refer to the mindless chatter as the "monkey mind"—you've likely heard that expression in a yoga class before. Before you immediately assign negativity to your churning thoughts, though, it's helpful to recognize that your mind reflects the natural state of the universe; that is, your mind is in perpetual movement (*vritti*) in the same way that the universe is. This ceaseless shifting of the larger world is *parinamavada,* and it is the basic state of all that is. Your mind is always learning, reconsidering, and questioning. While that may feel unmooring in moments, this constant changing reflects how things are in the universe at large. Recognizing that these fluctuations are normal—and also that you may want to bring more awareness and intentionality to your thoughts—allows you to approach yourself with compassion as you unpack the workings of your mind.

The Yoga Sutras tell us that there are five types of mind-shifts that regularly occur:

Pramana is right knowledge or comprehension. How marvelous it is to be a thinking creature! In our modern world, where you can conduct research on any topic that interests you via a cell phone, you are constantly broadening your understanding of the world, science, and humanity. We are in a state of constant learning, growing, and analyzing, and we can suddenly grasp key ideas about something we previously had no awareness of. Pramana refers to the full understanding of something or deep cognition. While you can rightly label this a fluctuation of your mind, it's not a bad one. After all, if your ideas don't evolve and your comprehension of the world doesn't grow, you find yourself in stasis, stuck with stagnant understanding and, likely, losing your wonder at the world.

Viparyaya is false knowledge or misapprehension. To be a thinking creature can also be challenging, when there are a host of political and social forces trying to sway your views on the world one way or another. When you seek knowledge but find yourself more confused—or worse, confident that the misinformation you've been misled into believing is true—that's viparyaya. This fluctuation of your mind is a much less helpful one. Modern technology has resulted in everyone having access to a microphone; everyone can easily share their thoughts or opinions, even when they are unhelpful, unkind, or worst of all, untrue. As a result, your mind may jump around from incorrect truth claim to incorrect truth claim, and you may ultimately wind up with the wrong idea about things.

Vikalpa means imagination. Not all imagining is bad! It's important to imagine a better world than the one you live in; that sort of hope can make it easier to live in a world of suffering. Imagination can also bring joy. How much fun is it as a child to imagine your dream home or design imaginary worlds? Vikalpa turns problematic and distracting when it casts forward, projecting catastrophe or creating anxious expectations about situations that have not yet come to fruition. When we imagine things that have not yet arisen, we can easily get consumed with events that may never even transpire. Imagination is not bad, but an unchecked imagining mind will certainly distract you from meditation and peace.

Nidra means deep sleep. In chapter 23, we'll talk about a specific form of yogic practice called *yoga nidra*. In this context, *nidra* is referring to the way your mind works on an unconscious level: essentially, dreams. Sometimes dreams can feel deeply important and resonant: You might see a friend or relative who has recently died, assuring you they are OK. But sometimes dreams can be nightmares, where your imagination takes you into places that your waking mind avoids.

Smrti is memory. Memories are important; you may notice that when you spend time with longtime friends, you almost immediately cast backward to reminisce on the "good old times." But if we spend too much time stuck in past memories—whether it's memories of when things were better or worse than they are now—it's neither helpful nor healthy. After all, the past is unchangeable. There's only so much time you should dwell on what was or what you did or what happened.

None of these movements of your mind are inherently bad. Even viparyaya, which we may want to avoid the most, also has its place. Sometimes not fully comprehending something creates magic (consider the joy of children who still believe in Santa Claus!), and sometimes we don't fully ascertain a situation out of a sense of self-preservation. (You may not want to know the full truth if knowing it will result in unnecessary suffering—as the expression goes, "ignorance is bliss.") Recognizing that your mind moves around in these five essential ways can help you better determine when you'd like to actively think and when you'd like to stay in the now.

ACTIONS

Label your mind's shifts. The goal is not to stop your mind's ceaseless shifting but to bring more awareness to it, so that you have more control over when and how this shifting occurs. This is especially the case if your shifting mind distracts you. For example, your anxious worries about the future might distract you from being present with your family, or your memories of the past might hinder your progression toward a better life. When your mind shifts, try to notice it. You may even imagine these shifts as physical locations: nidra might be a deep cave of murky images; smrti a movie theater with the past projected and flickering on a screen; vikalpa a great forest where there are amazing and terrifying creatures; viparyaya a maze where what you seek seems to be dashing around every corner, just in front of you; pramana an open, bright field of grass, where you can see far into the distance and you understand exactly what you're seeing. Notice when your mind is in the cave, the theater, the forest, the maze, or the field. Label those shifts and allow this labeling to bring you back to your mind, right here.

Write down your thoughts. The mind likes to ruminate. We bet that when you think of smrti, you'll realize that you're not being distracted by all your memories—you're being distracted by some *specific* memories. Have you written these memories down? Maybe your mind wants to play out the memories you have of a lost loved one. Writing this down will help you remember this loved one in greater detail, and it will allow you to let go of the fear of forgetting. Maybe you keep imagining a future event and attaching anxiety to it; can you write about it in two ways? First write down the event as you worry it will unfold: Your big speech lands flat and no one laughs at the lines you intend as jokes. But then write about this event again, letting your imagination bring you through the event as a successful, happy one, where things go as planned. You might imagine journaling to be something we do with a certain goal in mind, but in this action of writing down your thoughts, you're simply trying to give your thoughts somewhere else to go, so your mind can grow a little quieter.

5

KNOW THE DIVINE

What does yoga say about divinity? *Ishvara,* or divinity, is the most ancient of teachers, the manifestation of omnipotence, the seed of all consciousness. The divine is eternal, always. When we cultivate the right balance of indifference and presence, we tap into it and get a taste of it. The divine is also a broad enough concept to fit into either your understanding of faith or your humanistic worldview. You may see it embodied in the icons at church, in the gods on your home altar, or in the love you feel for your children or pets. You might experience the divine in nature on a hike at sunrise, or at sunset as you sit on the beach with a fruity drink.

We think reverence is an important guide. Reverence for the wonder of the world keeps you humble. It also helps you recognize that your stresses and woes, deadlines and detailed calendars, and quite often your everyday worries and anxieties are all for nought. In many cases, they are so unimportant in the grand scheme of all of existence as to be rendered nearly meaningless. That's not to say that they are meaningless to *you,* but by recognizing that not *much* matters when looking at the big picture of existence, you have the freedom of attaching less importance to them.

Your vision of the divine may be much more internal than external. One of our favorite American poets reminds us that our bodies are a constant reminder of divinity. In the poem "Song of Myself," Walt Whitman writes, "Divine I am inside and out, and I make holy whatever I touch or am touch'd from; / The scent of these arm-pits is aroma finer than prayer; / This head is more than churches, bibles, and all the creeds."[1] We've always loved this particular section of Whitman's writing. There is both humor and truth in remembering that we are divine creatures down to our stinky body odor. And this resonates with where we are now in Western yoga culture, which blossomed from the tantric embrace of the body as divine: Much of our modern-day yoga practice is about knowing the divine through the movement, choreography, and challenge of bringing yoga poses into fruition through your breath and life force. In this, your sense of divinity is expressed through your physical form.

While your vision of divinity doesn't have to be the same as Whitman's embodied divinity, we hope you arrive at a place where divinity feels personally resonant. That may take some investigating, uncovering, or immersion into mystical experiences—or a whole lot of yoga. We are but small, beautiful, bright spots of awareness and consciousness in an amazing, evolving, divine experiment. When you allow yourself to be in awe of the magic of existence, you sense the power of an extraordinary sunset, or feel God in the hymns of your congregation, or recognize the incredible nature of shared experience in a hug from your dearest friend. And in all these moments (and many, many more), you are knowing the divine.

ACTIONS

Make room for divinity, however you define it. To know the divine—inside and outside of yourself—set up intentional time to be present with that knowing. Wake up early to drink coffee on your porch with the sunrise, with no other aim than appreciating the beauty. Set aside time to dance to your favorite music with your children. Go to your yoga class with the intention of bearing witness to the beauty of your breath and body in movement, feeling the divine in the room as you settle into savasana.

Come back to spiritual ritual. When there are times in your life that you feel devoid of mysticism and unattached to the magic of being part of something greater, dive into experiences that might bring you back to wonder. Get up in the middle of the night to observe a meteor shower, attend kirtan (a chanting and singing practice common in yoga studios), read poetry, or stare at clouds. Build an altar in a sacred space in your house. Allow ritual experiences to harken to the divine.

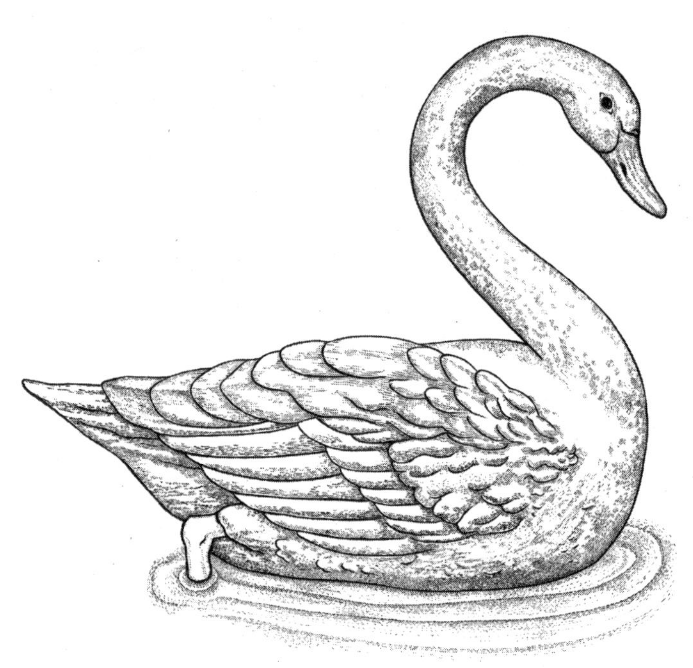

6

THE EIGHT LIMBS

The Yoga Sutras codify yoga knowledge and provide a system and a clear path to follow: We call it the "eight limbs." These practices are often seen as a ladder you climb up, rung by rung, to arrive at *samadhi*, ultimate bliss. But by now, you likely will have already experienced a taste of bliss (no ladder-climbing needed), or you wouldn't return to your yoga practice—or pick up a book like this. The eight limbs provide a path for the practice, not a ladder. This path includes asana, of course, but there is so much more to it than that. Here, we are condensing an explanation of these eight limbs down to a chapter, but they can be (and have been) the basis for entire books.

The first two limbs provide us five "don'ts"—the *yamas*—and five "dos"—the *niyamas.*

Yamas: The Abstentions (The Don'ts)

Yama means control or constraint. These are the *don'ts,* the things you should abstain from. You can consider them external observances, because they give you instructions for how to move in the world.

Because of this, others will be able to see whether or not you abide by the yamas. Following these principles will ensure that we get along as a society and build community with one another.

Ahimsa: *A-himsa* means nonviolence—the *a-* you see in most of these yamas, or don'ts, is a negative prefix. *Himsa* means harming—it's almost a cognate. The very first principle is to avoid violence and harm. This goes for how you relate to others and how you relate to yourself: Don't intentionally harm others and don't harm yourself. Live with the smallest "harm footprint" possible. Live with compassion for others and for yourself. We've already discussed how *atha* is arguably one of the most important words of the sutras. Combined with the very first yama, *ahimsa*, it becomes an essential directive: *Now, do no harm.* If that's as far as you get, it's good enough.

Satya: This word means "truth," and the directive to us is to be honest. Or, put another way, the directive is to be honest unless it will cause more harm than being dishonest. We love how this yama underscores the first one: "No, really; first, do no harm." We see it as an emphatic restatement of the prime directive of nonharming. It's also a reminder that moving through the world with honesty as a mandate is non-negotiable. It's a foundational aspect of yoga. Be honest with others. Be honest with yourself.

Asteya: Do not steal. (This is a direct cognate.) Stealing is a specific type of harm, taking things that are not rightfully yours. In our modern world, you probably don't steal items—but *asteya* is a reminder not to steal time or energy, either. Don't take more than is honestly yours. Don't take more than you need. Don't take anything that is not truly and rightly your own.

Brahmacharya: Brahma is the capital-S Self, the supreme life force, the divinity at the root of the universe. *Brahmacharya* means operating in a way befitting Brahma. Modern yoga interprets *brahmacharya* as meaning the responsible use of personal energy. In alignment with the renunciation inherent in the Yoga Sutras, from which this comes, you will sometimes hear this yama defined as "sexual chastity." We like the word *temperance* more: not complete abstinence but extreme moderation. It's the appropriate application of energy for the situation at hand, in alignment with the greater good. The better aware we are of the present, of the now, and the more we attend to the *now* where yoga takes place, the better we are able to bring the right energy to bear: not too much, not too little. Brahmacharya is responsible use of your personal energy: not using it to wantonly influence or harm others. This sense of temperance helps us balance between stealing, or taking what is not ours, and hoarding, or keeping back what we could give—the next yama.

Aparigraha: Here's that negative *a-* prefix again. *Aparigraha* means don't hoard; don't amass more than you need. Don't keep up with the Kardashians or the Joneses. Beware of spiritual salesmanship that pushes you to grasp for more than you need and to covet what others have. This is especially true in the practice of yoga, as capitalism tries to convince you that the *appearance* of enlightenment equals enlightenment itself!

When we commit to honest (satya) nonharming (asteya) and use the appropriate energy for the circumstances to act in alignment with the universal good (brahmacharya), we can find the right line between avoiding taking more than we need (asteya) and holding on to things we don't need (aparigraha). We think this is a pretty great directive for how to move through the world in a way that promotes harmony and well-being for yourself and others.

Niyamas: The Observances (The Dos)

Ni- is another negative prefix, like the *a-* in *ahimsa* and *asteya*. It also means "don't," and combined with *yama*, it creates a double negative: Don't not do this, do not control this. These niyamas are the dos, in contrast with the don'ts we saw in the yamas. While the yamas are about how we relate to other people—our external life—the niyamas are more about how we relate to ourselves—our internal life. Here, then, we already see the trip through the eight limbs as an inner journey, starting with how we walk in the world, and moving on to how we relate to ourselves. (Spoiler: The latter limbs continue this journey inward, and eventually we'll go even deeper to work on our connection to the divine within.)

Saucha: This is an injunction toward cleanliness. In older societies, before the hygiene advances of the modern era, this was critical for collective survival. Today, we like to think of it as paying attention to orderliness and minimizing the mess we create: in our relationships with others, in our domestic environments, and in the global environment. Be clean; leave no trace.

Santosha: This is an instruction for us to be happy—not in a surface "don't worry, be happy" or "good vibes only!" way, but to be happy despite whatever is going on around you. Find radical contentment with who you are, as you are, where you are. This is equanimity. Santosha is asking us to do what Wendell Berry (one of our favorite poets) exhorts in his poem "Manifesto: The Mad Farmer Liberation Front." He wryly (but sincerely) reminds us to "be joyful though you have considered all the facts."[1]

Radical contentment in the face of a "four a.m. wake-up, be productive, do-it-all" culture is an act of revolution. Hustle culture trains us to be comfortable with being uncomfortable—as do many versions of yoga asana, as presented in yoga studios. Santosha (and some of the sweeter styles of yoga that we love, like gentle, yin, and restorative yoga) teaches the opposite: comfort with comfort, being OK with just being OK. It means finding a way to be happy even as our institutions strain under harmful leadership or as harrowing world events unfold. This takes great effort. We fully understand that. You can think of santosha as a critical effort to make both personally and politically; after all, mindful joy is an act of resistance.

Tapas: Your fiery dedication and disciplined effort are *tapas*. You know it as the delicious freedom of discipline: freedom from choice. You go to yoga on Sunday mornings because that's what you do to stay committed to the practice. You wake up and meditate because it grounds you in your efforts of mindfulness. Tapas gives you the relief of knowing what to do and when to do it. We'll revisit this in future chapters as we continue to explore yoga's injunction to act without attachment to results.

Svadhyaya: This means self-knowledge, self-awareness, and self-study. You're doing this right now by reading this book! Svadhyaya can be interpreted both as study *on* your own, like homework, and study *of* your own self, a practice of self-knowledge and self-awareness. You see this bloom on the mat: Moments into savasana, an epiphany appears. In attempting a handstand, you learn about your perceived limitations. Svadhyaya is not just the unintentional self-knowledge you collect along the path of life—it's a recognition that part of your job on earth is to know yourself fully.

Ishvara Pranidhana: *Ishvara* is one of the names of the divine. This last niyama asks us to surrender to the recognition that there is something bigger than us all. Ultimately, let go. Saucha, tapas, and svadhyaya are all ways to *act* (even if that action is internal), while Ishvara pranidhana and santosha are ways to *be*. This means accepting what *is*, both materially (in the case of santosha) and universally (in the case of Ishvara pranidhana). Consider, too, that this act of surrendering and letting go is one of sweet relief. You are not in control. Phew!

Our favorite interpretation of these last three niyamas is one we learned from the yoga teacher Leslie Kaminoff. He suggests thinking of them in the sense of Reinhold Niebuhr's "Serenity Prayer," which you may know from its use in 12-step meetings: We are seeking the serenity to accept the things we cannot change (Ishvara pranidhana, surrender); the courage to change the things we can (tapas, dedication); and the critical wisdom to know the difference between the two (svadhyaya).

The yamas and niyamas serve as ethical guideposts for yogis, and they are probably familiar to you already. At the end of this chapter, we'll offer actions you can try to see how they can guide your life.

Asana

Since this book is about yoga *off* the mat, it's worth noting that yogic texts say very little about asana, the yoga poses. The sutras simply tell us that the seat, *asana*, should be both steady and comfortable—it should have elements of effort and elements of ease. Most early yogic texts don't mention physical poses or movements at all—or if they're mentioned, they're treated as a necessary part of creating comfort so that human bodies can sit comfortably in contemplation or meditation. Most of the poses that are central to a yoga practice these days—familiar shapes, like Warrior II—are inventions from the last 150-or-so years of yoga. Knowing that offers great freedom. It means that no pose is sacred. What's sacred is what you bring to it, what you learn from it, and how you use it as an opportunity for self-study.

Our modern-day movement practices and asanas give us a chance to practice physical balance. As we learn to find that sweet spot, whether it's in a vinyasa or a restorative yoga practice, we come to live even more in the present moment. Asana is a tool for balance and a tool to be in the now. You should move, and you can move in fancy ways, if you'd like. But ultimately, move in a way that allows you to better know yourself through movement.

Pranayama

Prana means the animating life force embodied by the breath. As we saw already, *yama* means control. So, one interpretation of *pranayama* is controlling (*yama*) the breath (*prana*). Another interpretation, put forth by T. K. V. Desikachar, is that there's a sneaky negative "*a-*" in there as an infix (in the middle of the word), the same negative we saw as a prefix for *ahimsa* and *asteya*. In this reading, *prana-a-yama* means removing any constraint of the free flow of prana. (We love this interpretation, as it emphasizes freedom and liberation!) Either way, we usually think of pranayama as breath practice. There are many different breath practices that are part of yoga. You may have encountered pranayama in the form of alternate-nostril breathing or lion's breath in a yoga class. There are many books available on breathing and breathwork. If that interests you, explore it!

At the heart of pranayama is this: Mindfully breathe. You can breathe in fancy, more complicated ways, if you'd like. But the most important thing is to breathe in *intentional* ways so that you may reconnect with your truest self through breath.

Pratyahara, Dharana, and Dhyana

Limbs five, six, and seven walk us through moving inward (*pratyahara*), concentrating and building focus (*dharana*), and meditating and cultivating presence (*dhyana*). The real work of yoga is in these limbs, where you build your ability to keep your awareness in the here and now. The real work of life is the internal work. You do that work best with space, peace, and quiet.

Pratyahara is the first step. It involves turning inward and tuning out the outside noise. That may be literal: You stay rooted in meditation, even as your child blasts the *K-Pop Demon Hunters* soundtrack in the next room. You remain in the present, even as it becomes obvious that someone burned toast at breakfast. You stay still and seated, even as you're aware that your left elbow feels itchy. The practice of pratayahara means you recognize these sense distractions, focusing on each of them, one at a time—and then you let them go. Pratyahara can be more evocative than literal. Perhaps the distraction you most need to let go of is the mental noise of the emails you have to send and the laundry you need to fold. Pratayahara can take form when you tune out the nagging voice that wants to needlessly review the past and preview the future. Instead, you go inward, to a space deep within you that is unaffected by what's happening outside.

Dharana means single-pointed concentration—your ability to focus on one thing, and only that one thing. You just did this by focusing on one sense at a time as you turned your attention inward. Keep going: Choose *one* thing you feel or think, or choose the rhythm of your breath, and then sustain your focus. It's harder than you might think. This is why yogis use tools like mantra (repeating a phrase) and drishti (setting your gaze): They help you sustain your attention on that one thing. Focus.

Once you're able to keep your attention on *one* thing, you can expand it again to include all the many things that are happening now: your breath, your thoughts, the light around you, the sound around you, and the immutable, unchanging *you*, here and now. This is *dhyana*, meditative awareness, or presence in the moment. It might feel like bliss, because it points to bliss: *samadhi*. (We'll go deeper into these ideas in chapter 7.)

Samadhi

Often, the harder you try to make something happen, the more elusive it can become. This is the case with *samadhi*, or complete and utter bliss. Instead of striving to arrive at samadhi as the end goal—instead of acting like there's any end goal at all—focus on the previous limbs. Control the controllables. See what happens. Remember, too, that although these limbs are sometimes presented as a ladder, they are not a set of rungs to climb that gets you to a certain goal at the top. Indeed, you've probably arrived at bliss through many (non-yogic) paths previously. (Chocolate cake comes to mind!) The eight limbs are a useful way to build more awareness and balance, which usually brings more joy. But there is no definite path to bliss, and the mystery and magic of the attainment of bliss are part of the wonder of existence.

ACTIONS

The eight limbs of yoga offer a map for finding the balance we already explored in chapter 3: the balance between stealing and hoarding; between fiery dedication and surrender; between effort and ease; between moving through the outer world and observing your inner experience; and between focus and presence. At the fulcrum of these balances is that sweet spot: samadhi.

Make decisions that honor balance. As you've seen, the yamas and niyamas are about walking in the world in ways that reduce harm and improve society. They encourage us to find the right balance between action and acceptance, between taking too much and holding back too much. They encourage us to be clean, be clear, and be kind.

The next time you're faced with a decision, consider how to make it with balance in mind. Start with a low-consequence decision, like what to eat for dinner, rather than whether or not to move cross-country! Filter this decision through the dos and don'ts that the yamas and niyamas lay out:

- Ahimsa: Where can I reduce harm?

- Satya: What is the truth here? How can I be honest?

- Asteya: Am I stealing from anyone as a consequence of this decision?

- Brahmacharya: What is the temperate thing to do here; what uses my energy most wisely?

- Aparigraha: Am I holding back something that I could be sharing?

- Saucha: What is the cleanest approach?

- Tapas: What can I do or give to make this decision happen, and what are its consequences or next steps?

- Svadhyaya: Given what I know of myself, what patterns or habits are contributing to my decision-making?

- Ishvara pranidhana: If this decision were out of my hands, if I surrendered this choice to the divine, where would I be guided?

Tune out, turn off, drop in. *Pratyahara* is often translated as "sensory withdrawal"—and that practice can be a shortcut to inner awareness. It involves the very opposite of the "Turn on, tune in, drop out" phrase Timothy Leary popularized in the 1960s, though the goal is the same: connection to the now.

Try it now: Notice what is coming in through your sense of sight. That could be these words you're reading (unless you're listening to the book in audio format); the page or the e-reader itself; and what's beyond that, including the quality of light in the room. Now tune out. Try softening your awareness, so you attend only to what's needed here and now. If that means closing your eyes for a few breaths, great!

Similarly, what is there to hear right now? Can you first increase your attention to everything your sense of hearing is offering? This could be sounds that are near to you or far away, or even sounds from within your body, like your breath, your digestion, or your heartbeat. Now can you turn off those sounds and turn your attention inward, so you're only hearing what's inside? And can you then soften that awareness?

Try something similar with your sense of smell and taste: Notice what you can notice, then soften that awareness. This leaves you with your sense of touch. Feel the book in your hands, your body sitting or reclining. Soften that awareness.

Now notice if any thoughts are serving as distraction. Go deeper—away from your senses, away from the chatter.

Now drop in. You're in the now. *Now begins the study of yoga.*

7

FLOW STATE

The Hungarian American psychologist Mihaly Csikszentmihalyi described "flow state" as something that happens when the ability of the practitioner and the challenge of the practice meet. He writes,

> *The best moments usually occur when a person's body or mind is stretched to its limits in a voluntary effort to accomplish something difficult and worthwhile. Optimal experience is thus something that we make happen.*[1]

We get to *dhyana*—the immersive meditative state we could call flow or presence—through the gateway of *dharana*, intense focus. And we come out the other side into *samadhi*, blissful connection. This is the surest path to samadhi. We can, however, sometimes be teleported in by the grace of the divine, or serendipity. The sutras say, "Some people just achieve samadhi," almost with a shrug at their luck. Sutra 1.19 is interpreted by a variety of authors to suggest that some people are innately "better" at yoga. For most of us, though, the path is dharana and dhyana.[2]

As we discussed in the previous chapter, the last of the eight limbs of yoga are concerned with meditation, focus, and attention. Have you had the experience of a state of focus elevating you to a state of joy? The more we spend time in this focused flow state, the more it becomes reflected in our outer-world experiences. Time spent in meditation or in a place of single focus allows us to become energetic, joyful, and understanding—and as a result, others might be more drawn to us. In sutra 1.25, we hear about the idea of *pratibhad va sarvam*, which means something like "intuitive knowledge"; essentially, this phrase means that the more you focus and flow, the more you'll be in a state of bliss, where wisdom will just innately flow to you.

The key is finding the right edge. If the task is overwhelming, you'll shut down. If it's underwhelming—if it's too basic for your abilities—you'll get bored and check out mentally. You need to find the "Goldilocks" sweet spot in which you experience both concerted effort and also a sense of ease. Some find this through exercise. Others find it through video games, or computer programming, or meditation.

ACTIONS

Choose where to spend your focus. You can't multitask well, despite your belief that you can! Instead, your focus and attention are a limited commodity that you should treat with care. Make purposeful, considered decisions about where to spend your energy. TikTok? Maybe not. Reading poetry? Maybe! When you sit down to work, put your phone face down. When you start to write an email, complete it before you jump tabs in your internet browser. In fact, close as many tabs of your browser as possible, so you're able to be pulled in to only the matter at hand. We've learned from being yoga teachers that attention has power. Many students come to class in order to be observed by someone who is facilitating and holding space for them. Attention is powerful. Don't give yours to media, people, or activities unworthy of it.

Challenge yourself near the limits of your ability. Find an activity that requires you to stretch yourself—one where you might even fail. Make it hard enough that there's some risk of not succeeding, but not so hard that it feels demoralizing. You may already do this in your yoga asana practice, but other physical practices can help you find this edge of your flow state: try Pilates or tai chi; take swimming or tennis lessons; learn to navigate a high ropes course. Or pick up a new habit that involves your hands and your brain: knitting, crochet, needlepoint, macrame, baking, canning, pickling, woodworking, pottery, jewelry making. The focus and presence needed to concentrate on learning new skills is yoga, a union of your attention and the present moment.

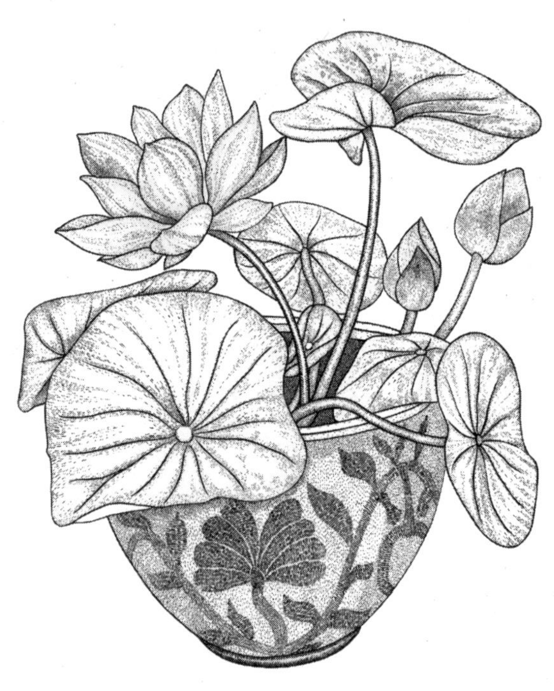

PART II

THE GOOD:
YOGA, HAPPINESS, AND POSITIVE PSYCHOLOGY

We practice yoga both on and off the mat because it brings us joy and connects us to a sense of divine meaningfulness. It can make your life better, and not just through movement. Yoga offers a way to expand your understanding of happiness and to live a more contented life. You've already learned about one way: *santosha*, or contentment, which we learned about in chapter 6. In part II, we'll walk through more of yoga's tools for enhancing the positive.

As we explore the technology of happiness, be careful of spiritual bypassing: the love-and-light, good-vibes-only approach that attempts to find a shortcut around the hard work of dealing with your negative feelings, personal traumas, and our collective hardships.[1] Spiritual bypassing cheapens spiritual practices by inverting them into a form of repression, misinterpreting "nonattachment" as a way to avoid processing difficult feelings. It is about closing off, using spiritual impulses to shut out truth, pain, or fear. Real spiritual processing requires seeing things as they are, attending to your fears, and finding healing for your pain.

As you read through part II, notice that the ideas here are about opening and expanding rather than contracting or hiding.

8

LIBERATION

Over the thousands of years of yoga's development, there have been plenty of changes to its philosophy. At certain points, the practice was very esoteric, rejecting the physical body and teaching that liberation could be achieved through the renunciation of the material realm. At other points, the physical body was embraced as an important spiritual vehicle for freedom. But despite these fluctuations, liberation has always remained a primary aim of yoga.

We love having liberation as a spiritual aim. Yoga's goal is not repentance or forgiveness or (at this point in time) renunciation; it's simply for you to find freedom. Isn't that a gloriously happy goal?

Even better, yoga shows us that you achieve this goal not by making yourself smaller in the face of the divine but by remembering that you are *part* of the divine. What a joyful message: Liberation is simply recalling your own innate sacredness!

We spoke in the previous chapter about the path of the eight limbs, the last of which is samadhi, or bliss. That's one way to think about liberation: You can practice all aspects of yoga, and you're likely to find your way to bliss. But one thing we love about yoga's concept of liberation is that you can also arrive there by *realizing you've already arrived.*

Consider this: You've already experienced true and complete freedom. Think of a time when you've felt most at peace, at ease, at one. Maybe it was a particular moment of family bliss on a vacation to a gorgeous, vista-laden destination. Maybe it was snuggling in bed with a good book and a mug of something warming. Maybe it was being alone in your home, marinating in the silence surrounding your breath. You've certainly felt it at least a few times at the end of savasana in yoga. (We bet that's one big reason you've returned to yoga: that very feeling of liberation, that realization that the divine is already in you.)

That's the magic: In most of these cases, you didn't have to do much or anything at all to arrive at liberation. Perhaps you had the right frame of mind to notice it. Maybe you had the emotional or physical space to recognize it. But you didn't really *do* anything to create your own liberation. You didn't have to journey there. That's because there is no difference between the journey and the destination. You are liberated through your recognition of your liberation.

ACTIONS

Don't try to grasp the fish. Recognizing your liberation is like catching a fish with bare hands: The fish is wriggly and slippery, and it's nearly impossible to hold onto it for long. Imagine, then, that you're not trying to hold onto liberation; instead, you're trying to find fleeting glimpses of it. You're not fishing to catch a fish but rather to observe its wonders: its scales, its muscles, the gorgeous way it glides through water.

Choose a mantra. To bring yourself back to this experience of observing your liberation, you can create a mantra—a phrase or word—that encompasses what previous moments of liberation have felt like for you.

Maybe your word or phrase is deeply unique to you and your experiences, but you can also play with Sanskrit words that evoke the idea of liberation—words like *moksha*, *nirvana*, and *kaivalya*. These words are threaded through yoga philosophy. *Moksha* comes from the Upanishads (sometimes called Vedanta, or literally, the end of the Vedas) and suggests the specific liberation of recognizing self and divine are the same—in this context, the union of Atman and Brahman. *Nirvana*, the liberation of being released from suffering, is common in the Buddhist tradition. *Kaivalya* comes from the Yoga Sutras, where it points to liberation as discerning Self (*purusha*) as distinct from matter (*prakriti*). Maybe one of these words, with their subtle differences in liberation, is especially evocative for you. Create your liberation mantra to reconnect to what you already know.

What is freedom? Another helpful practice when considering liberation is to define it for yourself. What makes you feel least restricted or subjugated? Maybe it's waking up to a day that has no plans at all. Or maybe it's waking up to a day that has perfectly considered plans already in place, down to reservations and transportation. For different people, one of these scenarios may feel like bliss while the other feels confining. This underscores that freedom has a different flavor for everyone. Within the circumstances that are under your control, how can you create more opportunities for experiencing freedom in your life?

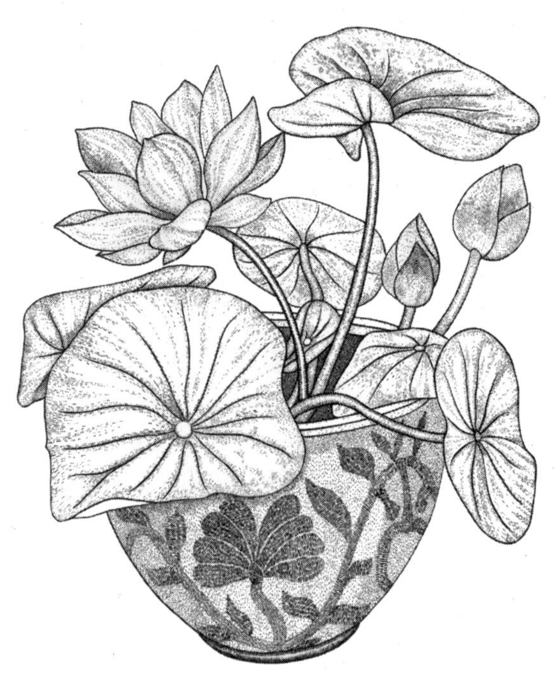

9

COMPASSION

Metta is a Pali word meaning loving-kindness or compassion toward all beings—including ourselves. While you might imagine compassion as an active practice, it's actually a little more complex. Showing up in empathy and compassion means being attentive and present to someone else's suffering, but it doesn't (necessarily) mean fixing or solving that suffering. Compassion means holding space for someone else's pain. The only active part is this: You must hold space while *withholding* judgment. While that may be the harder part, it is at the heart of why we practice.

As you certainly know, if you want to get better at something, you have to practice. Whether it's playing a piano piece or running a 5K at a particular pace, you can't just *say* you want to get better at it. You have to put in the time, effort, and commitment. Likewise, you must practice to build your compassion and loving-kindness. You have to practice offering compassion without judging those who are suffering.

Enter metta meditation, a practice from the Buddhist tradition that is often offered in yoga, too. We find metta meditation to be one of the sweetest and most accessible practices in all of yoga, and it's worth doing daily. Metta meditation is a reminder that to exist is to suffer. In metta meditation, you will send good wishes of loving-kindness toward yourself, your loved ones, neutral people, difficult people, and all beings—since suffering is a universal experience. The practice is to send these good wishes without judgment or attachment to outcomes or change. You freely offer love with no other intention than offering love.

ACTIONS

Practice metta meditation. Make yourself comfortable, whether you're sitting, reclining, or moving. Pull up the image of a loved one in your mind. This can be a parent, a child, a sibling, a romantic partner, a dear friend, or a pet. They may be living or deceased; just imagine them as clearly as you can. Perhaps you can imagine how this dear one smells or sounds, or how it feels to hug or pet them. (If this gets you emotional, you're doing it right!) Practice sending metta, loving-kindness, to this beloved: *May you be happy. May you be healthy. May you be whole.* If you have time, choose another loved one and keep going, sending love and compassion to the dearest beings in your life.

Next, think of someone neutral—the cashier at the market, someone you might see walking down the street, or the person nearest your mat in your last yoga class. Pull up as good an image of them as you can. Then practice sending them loving-kindness: *May you be happy. May you be healthy. May you be whole.* If you have time, continue to send compassion to other people you know, but not well—for example, the parents of your friends or similar people that you are aware of, but to whom you do not routinely give much thought.

In the third step of this meditation, you'll send loving-kindness to yourself. (Some teachers *begin* with sending metta to yourself, but we find it's easier when you are warmed up, just like reps at the gym or intervals on the track.) Picture yourself as though you were looking in the mirror, or imagine your favorite picture of yourself—one in which you're happy and smiling. Send yourself loving-kindness: *May I be happy. May I be healthy. May I be whole.* If you have time to keep going, imagine yourself as a child, as a friend, as a coworker, as a parent, or as a lover; visualize yourself in your best moments and in your hardest, and send metta to every version and aspect of yourself.

Now that you're warmed up, take the time to choose someone you find difficult. Don't pick your mortal enemy or a world leader that deservedly inspires ire, but instead start with someone you find mildly irksome. Picture this person as clearly as you can. If you feel a physical reaction, notice that. Take a deep breath and offer yourself compassion again as you try to neutralize that reaction. Now send this difficult person loving-kindness, too. You do not have to like them, but you have to find the space to see them as a being that experiences suffering, too, and who is thus worthy of compassion: *May you be happy. May you be healthy. May you be whole.* You may need to repeat this part of the meditation a few times, until your heart means it. Over time, as you practice this meditation, this portion may include more than one challenging person. But beginning with one is a good place to start.

Finally, imagine all of the recipients of your goodwill arrayed before you—your loved ones, your community members, yourself, those who are challenging—and send them *all* your loving-kindness. *May we all be happy. May we all be healthy. May we all be whole.*

To hear a guided version of this meditation, head to www.sage rountree.com/yogaoffthemat.

Live metta meditation. Once you're familiar with metta meditation, you can layer it onto your other activities to squeeze in more practice. Send metta to a different person during each round of your sun salutations, or each quarter-mile of your run, or each pause for sniffs as you walk the dog, or each dish you wash, or each stoplight that's red. The more you practice, the better you will become!

10

ANOTHER WAY TO SEE THINGS

Pratipaksha bhavana—called "cognitive reappraisal" in therapeutic or psychological environments—is a reminder to try different ways of looking at things. Often in life, your own view is limited; you may be missing critical pieces of information that would explain how others are acting. (As we will explore in part III, the related teaching of *avidya,* or wrong-seeing, points to this as the primary cause of suffering.) When you feel the temptation to judge kicking in, or when your frustration begins welling up or bubbling over, take the time to posit a few alternative explanations for why someone is doing what they are doing. This can be as simple as thinking, "Maybe that driver is having trouble with their contact lenses, and that is why they are going so slowly," or as complicated as, "What if this whole situation had nothing to do with me, and if others' actions were not a statement about my own worth?" Or its opposite: "What if this whole situation is happening because of my *own* actions—what if *I'm* the unintentional bad guy here, instead of the martyred victim?"

Taking a situation and flipping it is a practice in flexibility off the mat. It parallels what we do when we practice asana on the mat: We take a situation and turn it in space to see what changes. Staff pose, downward-facing dog, and boat pose are all the same fundamental shape as legs up the wall, but each of them puts your body in a different relationship to gravity. As a consequence, each requires different loads on your core, shoulders, hamstrings and hip flexors, and nervous system. By taking the same basic shape—a lengthened spine and legs, combined with hip flexion—and turning it, we see the experience arrange itself differently, like a kaleidoscope. Similarly, the act of pratipaksha bhavana can both ease your suffering and build your compassion—two of the chief goals of yoga.

ACTIONS

Look back—way back—with perspective. There are probably several circumstances from your youth that, with time and experience, you now realize you misunderstood. The breakup you took so personally may prove in hindsight to really have been worthy of the "it's not you, it's me" line that you thought rang hollow at the time. The insult that once stung may feel different now, given the work you've done to acknowledge and correct your previous deficiencies. The rules your parents enforced when you were a child that felt so stultifying might seem perfectly reasonable now that you are a parent yourself.

With the buffer of time, you might be able to reappraise these situations with dispassion. See if you can untangle the truth hidden in the stories that we layer over what's really happening.

Brainstorm some alternative narratives. Take a more recent situation that you found mildly irksome. Brainstorm as many alternative narratives as you can. What might have really been going on that you knew nothing about, since you had only a slice of the facts surrounding the situation? It's OK to get silly, like "Maybe that wasn't my sister at all but an alien masquerading as her. Or maybe a witch put me under a spell that made me *think* it was her. . . ." As you brainstorm these alternative narratives, consider how you can view yourself and others through metta, or compassion. If you know someone who hurt you was similarly suffering, does it change the situation and your anger over it? Envisioning various scenarios as a way to explain things will defuse your frustration with others' behavior. As you imagine these alternatives, you'll recognize that your initial understanding of events was not the correct or only perspective. There's always another way to see things.

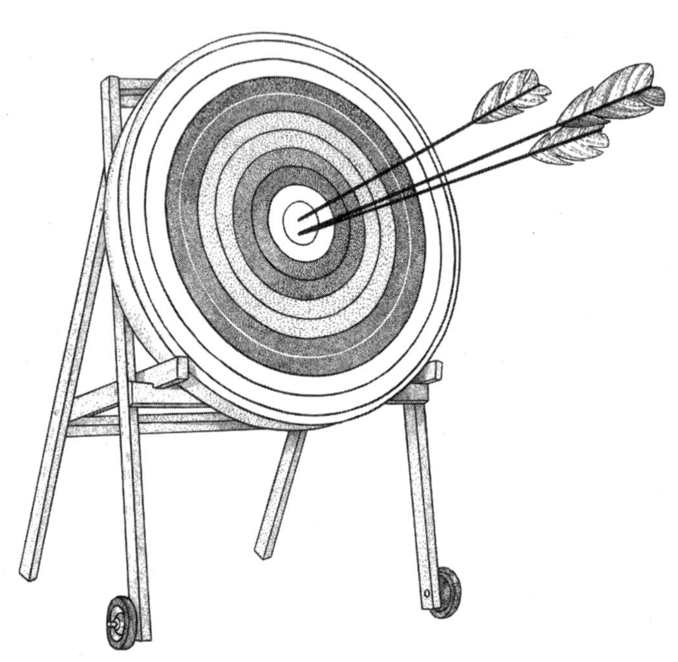

11
YOUR HIGHER PURPOSE

Hatha yoga and the modern practice of physical poses is just one variety of yoga; others include bhakti and karma yoga. As the yoga of devotion, bhakti yoga helps us center the divinity we find behind the poses. That might look like chanting, attending kirtan, going to church, or creating an altar. We know a yoga teacher who is steeped in the bhakti tradition, and he practices by following the teachings of the modern-day "hugging saint," Mata Amritanandamayi, better known as Amma. In karma yoga, we connect to the higher purpose of helping others, caring for our fellow travelers on the journey. Sometimes this manifests as offering free or discounted yoga classes for an under-privileged or historically disenfranchised population. Through selfless service, we come to see the humanity in everyone and, ideally, remove some of the barriers that stand between us and liberation.

Both bhakti and karma yoga practices involve letting go of our self-focus and turning our interest and efforts toward others: the divine (bhakti yoga) and other people (karma yoga). We imagine that in your most generous moments, you want the fruits of your actions to serve others. You recognize that you are a divine being on a planet of divine beings—and even in our divinity, we need support and kindness. That's the essence of both bhakti and karma yoga, taking that recognition of the divine and allowing your yoga to spring from devotion and service.

ACTIONS

Find ways to be of service. This could mean finding ways to volunteer in your community, but it can also mean smaller, daily acts of kindness, like paying a compliment to your barista, letting someone with fewer items and a child in tow cut in front of you at the grocery checkout, or picking up roadside litter and putting it in the trash. Karma yoga may already be present in your livelihood—maybe you're in a helping profession (like yoga or healing arts), and helping others feels like an effortless part of your being. Finding ways to be of service may be a new experience to you, though, and that's OK, too. Karma yoga asks us to be of use to others, to support them, and to help. How can you bring more of that into your life?

Find ways to praise. This is a great use of your social-media time. Instead of engaging in a pile-on or leaving snarky comments, share and praise what is good. Even if it's a cat video that brings a smile to your face, that's a manifestation of the divine and worthy of praise! Sometimes it seems like the internet is a place to compete for the most intellectual retort or the sickest burn. Could your time on social media be an opportunity to see the divine in others and share your divine light?

12

JOY

You may have heard the common saying, "Comparison is the thief of joy." This quote is so beloved and widely shared because it resonates deeply. From our earliest days, and then with increasing intensity from middle school onward, we allow comparing ourselves to others to steal our contentment, our bliss, and our connection to our own true, joyful selves.

Never do we feel this more than when we're perusing the infinite feeds on our social media. There is no bottom to the scroll, and no bottom to the depth of despair that we create for ourselves when we obsessively compare ourselves to the glossy sheen that others project on their social-media feeds.

Maitri is a concept from the Upanishads that is related to metta, or loving-kindness. The words share a root: *mid*, meaning love. When we practice delight in others' delight, we are engaging in maitri. We align our happiness with others' happiness. This is easy to do with your loved ones, but it's hard to do with your frenemies on social media. There, we more often engage in feeling bad about others' happiness. We compare ourselves, deem ourselves unworthy, and create our own suffering. Or maybe we indulge in the opposite: *schadenfreude,* a word taken from German that means feeling happy about others' sadness or misfortune. It makes us feel high to see someone brought low.

Either way, the state of comparison puts us out of alignment: One person is happy, the other is sad. In maitri, we are in alignment: Our happiness is a reaction to the happiness of others. We are best aligned when we delight in the delight of others, experience joy from their joy. At the other end of the spectrum, when another is sad and we are sad in reaction, we are in a state of compassion. Sometimes that's a lovely resonance, and sometimes it's uncomfortable. When we feel icky about someone else's suffering, Mexican-Spanish uses the term *pena ajena.* It roughly translates, in today's vernacular, to "cringe"— feeling embarrassment at the shame of others.

Consider the four-quadrant grid here. Your own simplified feeling—sad or happy—rests on one axis, and others' feelings of sadness or happiness on the other.

	THEY FEEL SAD	THEY FEEL HAPPY
I FEEL HAPPY	schadenfreude	maitri
I FEEL SAD	compassion/cringe	useless comparison/creating my own suffering

To experience yoga, union, and connection, we need to be aligned with others. Notice how when we delight in others' misfortune, or feel sad about their *good* fortune, we are in a state of disconnection and bad alignment. This evokes the term *dukha,* which literally means "bad axle space." On a wheel, this kind of misalignment of the axle space will wear down the wheel faster than when it has a better-aligned axle hole.

When our internal state reflects what the other is experiencing— whether it's that we are both happy, or we are both sad—we are *in* alignment. And this is where yoga happens: in the union between the personal experience and the universal, the experience of you as the subject and the other as the object.

Armed with this knowledge, you can take a new approach. Scrolling through social media is the perfect time to practice maitri, happiness in others' happiness. The more you practice, the easier it becomes, so practice celebrating every chance you get. What will eventually kick in with regular practice of maitri is an anti-comparison. You'll start to be happy that others are happy, because they show that this happiness is a possibility. You'll be happy that others are successful, because they show that this success is a possibility. And you'll start to see that these things are possible for you, too.

ACTIONS

Here are a few practical tips for how to do this when engaging with social media:

Double-tap everything. Love it all—and mean it. Try saying it out loud: "Yay, you!" (This builds on the bhakti yoga action from the previous chapter.)

"Good for her!" You may have seen the meme of Lucille Bluth, the matriarch character on *Arrested Development*, saying "Good for her!" In the context of the show, she says this after watching a news report saying a woman has driven her car into a lake on purpose, fed up with the patriarchy. While the original scene is ironic, this is another affirmation you can practice when you see others taking action and doing what's right for them: "Good for her!"

Take comfort in connection. As you'll learn in part III, *avidya*, wrong-seeing, is the root of suffering. When we feel jealousy, envy, or comparison, we are operating under the wrong-seeing presumption that we are separate from the objects of our feelings. By celebrating others' joy, we get to align our feelings with theirs, to resonate with them, and to connect—even if it's only through a screen. That connection increases everyone's joy!

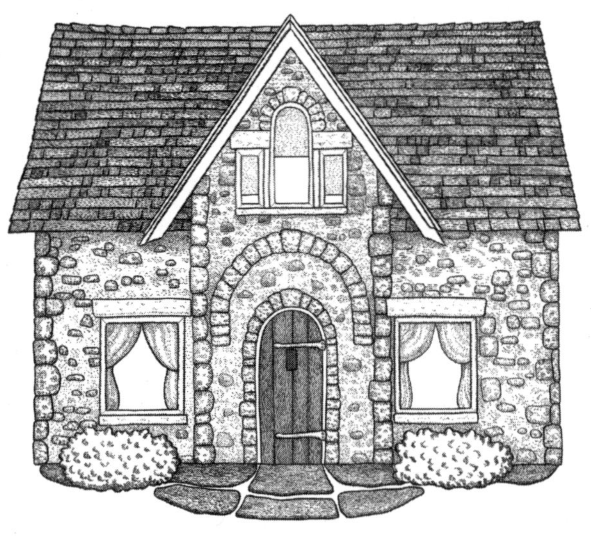

13

DIVINE PLAY

In tantric yoga, *spanda* is the pulse of life, the vibration that underlies all of existence; it reminds us that consciousness is dynamic and ever-changing. *Lila* is this divine consciousness at play; it shows us the creative, joyful, and spontaneous unfolding of the universe. Children tap into this sense of play, seamlessly immersing themselves fully in whatever activity or plan is happening and then leaving it behind to move onto other things. As adults, we can tap into our sense of play through improv, ecstatic dance or yoga dance, free movement, singing, or other activities that bring us joy.

Lila is a reminder that yoga can be resolute without being serious. A sense of lightness keeps you from taking yourself too seriously; being able to see the humor in things allows you to move without caring about how you look. It allows us to stumble, even to fall, and to get back up with a smile.

ACTIONS

Get out of your comfort zone. Try out a partner-yoga class or a laughter-yoga class. Or create your own spontaneous and unserious experience by throwing yourself a dance party. Put on your favorite songs and let your body move. Children are usually great partners for this—their lack of self-consciousness is inspiring. This type of silly letting go isn't just an important part of existing with joy; it's an important way to know yourself and trust yourself. In our yoga-teacher training, trainees are thrust into an evening of improv with a skilled improv teacher. While there is initially a sense of uncertainty among the trainees, this night of spontaneous silliness is often remembered as one of the best parts of training. In our very serious world, it's easy to forget that your true nature is playful. Try new things to remind yourself.

Watch a standup-comedy special. This doesn't mean watching your favorite reruns of *The Office*, but something fresh by a comic who's new to you. The novelty is part of the play. Comedy thrives on delivering on expectations via predictable patterns, but also on pattern disruption. When you engage with a story that you think you know, but something unexpected happens, you're put more fully in the moment: You delight in this surprise through laughter. And that is the *now* where yoga happens.

Attend kirtan or drumming. If your area offers collective chanting or drumming experiences, try them! Joining your voice or drumming in rhythm with others is a powerful way to be in the moment while tapping into the divine play of music. Riff a little; try a new note, a run, a syncopation. This is the divine expressing itself through you!

PART III

YOGA AND THE SHADOW SELF:
THE KLESHAS AND OTHER THINGS THAT HOLD US BACK

So far in this book, we've talked a lot about freedom and liberation. That raises the question: *Freedom from what?* What are we trying to disentangle and free ourselves from? Yoga has many answers to this question. The *kleshas*—referred to as the causes of suffering or the five obstacles to full realization—are impediments to the full experience of yoga. The five kleshas are *avidya* (wrong-seeing), *asmita* (ego), the twins of *raga* and *dvesha* (attachment or craving and aversion) and *abhinivesha* (the fear of the ultimate unknown). We'll discuss these concepts in depth in these next chapters. But it's not just the kleshas that hold us back; in general, yoga philosophy teaches us that getting stuck and ceasing to evolve can add suffering to existence.

We'll consider two key ideas to help explain this: *samskara* (ruts) and *vasana* (impressions). Another important concept is *maya*, or the illusion of separateness. Understanding these parts of yoga philosophy gives you tools to move through life with less unnecessary suffering.

14

WRONG-SEEING

The root of our suffering is so often in our misunderstanding, misperception, or misinterpretation of things: *avidya*. In imagery that depicts all five kleshas together, avidya is often given the form of the broad trunk of a tree, with the other four kleshas extending from it as branches. That's because misperception or wrong-seeing is at the heart of the other kleshas, too. Remember the *a-* from the yamas *ahimsa*, *asteya*, and *aparigraha*? Here it combines with the Sanskrit word for vision and sight, *vidya*. As fallible humans, we almost never have the full picture; we are always looking at the world and events in our lives through the lens of our own experiences, hurts, needs, and wants, which distorts our vision. Wrong-seeing is the status quo—it's the default nature of things. And this creates suffering.

As we saw in chapter 10 with pratipaksha bhavana, there is always an alternative explanation of what could be going on in any situation; there is always another way to look at things. This is why cognitive reappraisal and compassion are so important. But like many things, the wrong-seeing itself is neutral. It becomes negative only when we attach ourselves to it, when we cling to it and tell ourselves it is the truth.

You may know the parable of the blind men and the elephant: When encountering an elephant for the first time, each of them receives a limited understanding of what an elephant is depending on what part of its body they touch. An elephant could seem like a tree if you are touching only its leg, or a snake if you are touching only its tail or its trunk, or a wall if you're touching only its flank, or a spear if you're touching only its tusk. Each of these is a limited picture of the whole. While each one is not wrong, none of them are entirely correct. These individual perceptions are actually misperceptions, and to extrapolate from one part creates a misunderstanding of the whole picture. That's avidya.

If we get too attached to the limited view we have of any proverbial elephant, then we are creating suffering—ours and probably others'—by keeping our field of focus too narrow to see the larger truths.

ACTIONS

Question, and question again. Inspired by "The Work" of Byron Katie, here is an exercise to help you root out wrong-seeing. If you're not familiar with Katie's "four questions," we recommend her book *Loving What Is* for context; this is a focus on the first two questions, "Is it true?" and "Can I absolutely *know* it is true?"

When you find yourself confronted by a problem or frustration, take some time to consider the "facts" of the situation as you see them. Then ask: "Is it true?" You'll probably think, "Well, yeah, that's why I'm frustrated!" As we suggested in chapter 10, the work is then to go deeper and question yourself: "Can I absolutely *know* it is true?" Here, the answer is usually, if not always, *no*. Try to identify the assumptions that you are likely making based on both your own history and biases and your limited view of the facts of the situation at hand. Posit alternative explanations for what might be happening. Imagine zooming out to get the bigger picture, taking into account other possibilities. Draw your focus off the wrong-seeing and redirect it to the right-seeing.

Practice right-seeing. Deepen your exploration of the nature of reality by becoming curious about the reality of nature. Take time in the forest or a meadow to really investigate what you see from every angle. Don't just look at a flower from the path, step off the trail and look at it from the top, from the side, and from underneath. Use the magnification feature on your phone or camera—or an actual magnifying lens—to zoom in and see the elements that make up the flower. Notice the veining of the petal, the stamen or carpels, the variety of colors, and how these elements relate to each other.

Paying attention to this level of nuance and detail is a reminder that every situation has a lot more going on than you might immediately clock at first glance. Learning to pay attention this deeply will increase your ability to see clearly and decrease your suffering from wrong-seeing. This sort of mindful awareness and curiosity about nature has the added bonus of keeping you in the moment and enriching your appreciation for the divine world around you!

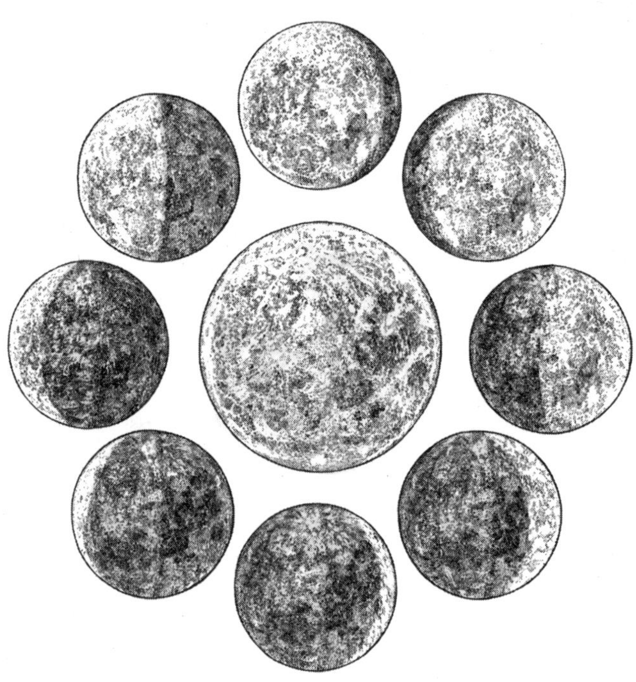

15

EGO

Second only to wrong-seeing is the suffering caused by your ego, *asmita*. As we noted in the previous chapter, the branches and leaves of ego grow from the tree of misperception. Attachment to ego is caused by the idea that you are separate from everyone and everything else. Your ego is deeply concerned with self-protection, self-importance, and self-preservation. When you recognize that your ego is striving to keep you safe and stay in control (even though that control is an illusion!), it's a little easier to have empathy for your ego-driven moments—and to shift away from ego-driven habits.

When you're identifying with your ego, you're identifying with your small-s self instead of your big-S Self—the universal Self. Your small-s self is consumed with vanity, pride, and hubris, generally in comparison to others. Your small-s self is concerned with having enough and often sees the world through the lens of scarcity, believing that there are not enough resources (whether that's food, money, love, time, or something else) for everyone to have enough and be satiated. In the modern world, we see a lot of unchecked ego-driven activity, as well as the suffering it leaves in its wake. This is where we may remind you that although this book is about how yoga philosophy can help you personally, the heart of yoga is not apolitical. When you look at all the elements we present in this book, it's obvious that in order to live in a way that is compassionate and yogic, your political choices have to arise from compassion and yoga, too.

With ego, you're blinded to the reality of the large-S Self that is all of us, connected. In chapter 20, we'll talk more about *maya*, the illusion of disconnection at the heart of ego. Ego tells you you're separate from others, when the reality is that you are part of the whole. Ego tells you you're more important than others, when the reality is that you and others are equally important, because we are all inextricably connected. Ego would have you forget that another's suffering is your suffering, too. Ego creates imaginary walls and unnecessary division. Asmita gets in the way of your ability to walk in the world from a place of true yoga. This echoes the fluctuations of the mind, the *chitta vritti*, that get in the way of yoga, too. When you successfully calm these fluctuations and move away from identifying with your petty ego, you rest in the peace of your true nature: a piece of the divine whole.

It's all too easy to get attached to your ego, because it is the lens through which you see virtually everything. Ego is not quiet or complacent. On the contrary, your ego is like a very loud and persistent toddler who only can speak one word: *me.* Imagining your ego as a whiny child can help you bring empathy to your ego-driven self— and to others' ego-driven selves! After all, asmita comes from a place of fear: fear that there is not enough, that you are not enough, that your needs won't get met, that you will be hurt. Recognizing that fear can allow you to soothe that needy-baby ego, offer it nurturing, and help it see its deep connection to everything and everyone around it.

ACTIONS

Loving self-callout. Recognize when you are operating from an attachment to ego. Consider moments in which you feel emotionally threatened, are trying to "save face," or are focusing on your appearance or how others perceive you. Lovingly call yourself out on it: "My ego is not my Self." One reminder here comes from Walt Whitman's "Song of Myself": "Do I contradict myself? / Very well then I contradict myself, / (I am large, I contain multitudes.)"[1] Whitman reveals that the true Self lives beyond the petty identifications of the ego and is large enough, multitudinous enough, to hold contradictory opinions at the same time—after all, the true Self is everything, all of us.

View your life as a movie/TV show. Another word for overattachment to ego comes from the Greeks: *hubris*. You likely remember that hubris, excessive pride, has been the downfall of tragic heroes since the beginning of storytelling. Icarus's elation at his flying skills led him to fly too close to the sun, despite his father's warnings; his wax wings melted, and he crashed. Heroes (and anti-heroes) in modern stories, too, let their ego get the better of them, leading them to their tragic fates—think Walter White in *Breaking Bad*, Daenerys Targaryen in *Game of Thrones*, or Elsa in the throes of her power in *Frozen*.

Take a cue from these dramatized examples and watch yourself as you would watch a character on a screen. Notice where an overidentification with ego tips into hubris that would lead to your eventual comeuppance if you were in a fictional story. Imagine how a situation might look to an outside viewer. Would they be yelling at the screen or booing and throwing popcorn? If you were watching, would you be able to easily identify the main character's folly? If so, you're probably acting from ego at that moment!

Dance like no one is watching. Much of our attachment to ego comes from thinking about how others will perceive us. Who are you when there's no one to see? Is that closer to the "real" you, to the light inside of you? Can you take that version of you out on the town and dance like no one is watching? That is, can you express your true nature in a variety of life situations, without attachment to others' perceptions of you? Although it can initially feel uncomfortable, this practice of vulnerability is a good way to quiet the ego and let your truest Self shine bright.

16

CRAVING AND AVERSION

Two of the kleshas are the two sides of one coin: craving (*raga*) and aversion (*dvesha*). These obstacles to your true freedom are connected to the other kleshas, as well; the coin of raga and dvesha is minted from avidya, wrong-seeing, and then polished by attachment to ego, asmita.

Raga and dvesha create suffering because they cause you to pay undue attention to the push and pull of what you feel you want and don't want. When there is a lot of emotional weight placed on your "likes" and "dislikes," you are made vulnerable to the vicissitudes of life, since quite often getting something you want or avoiding something you dislike is outside of your control. Consider what craving and aversion are: Craving is wanting something that isn't here to be available—and stat! That could be chocolate, sex, entertainment, or any of the hedonic pleasures. Aversion is wanting something that *is* here, like a bad feeling or pain, to go away. That could be boredom, physical pain, heartbreak, or any other manner of unpleasantries.

While craving and aversion may show up in response to serious, challenging life events, like an unexpected death of a loved one or a job loss, they are omnipresent in smaller, daily interactions with the world. This could be things like impatience while waiting in traffic, the frustrations of parenting, or an incorrect lunchtime order. Raga shows up when you feel upset because your usual latte order isn't made the way you want. Dvesha shows up in the frustration of having to sit and do your taxes. It's useful to recognize how your attachment and antipathy to small moments of life create suffering that could easily be avoided. Both craving and aversion are an act of fighting the reality of things *as they are*. In craving or attachment, you are trying to pull in something you don't have; in aversion, you're pushing away what you do have but don't want. Both struggles cause suffering because they are fighting the truth of what is real in the immediate moment.

The more you practice radical acceptance and right-seeing of what is actually true in the here and now, the less you will suffer the whims of your desires and revulsions.

ACTIONS

How can we increase our comfort with things just as they are, while decreasing our identification with our desires? We do it by taking small steps.

A mindful pause. When you feel a craving (whether it's for wine, chocolate, TV, or your correct and perfect latte order), stop and take a deep breath. Do it again. And again, if you can. Sometimes three breaths taken with awareness can remind you that you are experiencing a temporary drive to consume this thing. Noticing that can soften the desire, the craving, and the suffering it leaves in its wake.

Delay with a benign placeholder. Instead of insisting you won't give in to your craving, could you first try something more benign? When you feel a craving for an alcoholic drink, for example, could you first have a mocktail or kombucha—maybe even in a lowball or a wine glass? When you feel a craving for sweets, could you first eat a piece of fruit? When you want to watch television, could you instead sit in your TV-watching chair, lean back, and put your feet up, while the TV stays off? If your craving continues, you can return to it in twenty minutes or so, but sometimes these benign placeholders scratch the itch for what we wanted enough to let the craving pass.

Mild exposure therapy. Many of our aversions are so deeply ingrained that they become knee-jerk reactions: We smell something foul and recoil, we spot a spider and cringe. In safe circumstances, a mild amount of exposure therapy—intentional engagement with the stress stimulus that repels us—can condition us to abide even in circumstances where we either once experienced or currently feel aversion.

One classic example is for the snake-averse person to visit the reptile hall at the zoo, where the snakes are safely behind glass. Another is for the anxious introvert to go to the park, sit down on a bench by a stranger, and strike up a conversation. There's no need to face your deepest fear all in one go, but intentional exposure to uncomfortable situations will quickly build your confidence in your ability to handle them. This is mindful presence in action: You're consciously *choosing* to be here, now, in this (uncomfortable) moment, regardless of what you wish were here or weren't here. You're seeing things as they are, right here, right now. And when you do that, you're resting in your true nature.

Recognize that disinclination is formed of habit. Strong dislikes and aversions may not even be connected to reality as it is; sometimes our present aversion is based on a past event or impression. That aversion can become a habit that needs to be changed. When Alexandra's daughter rode a rollercoaster for the first time, the result was a lot of tears. For many years after that, she was deeply averse to all amusement rides, citing this first (scary!) experience.

That aversion became an ingrained habit. As children do, she grew bigger and older, and her likes and dislikes shifted. Years later, she tried riding the same roller coaster again and was amazed at how much fun it was! Similarly, you probably have aversions based on past experiences that may no longer hold sway over you. When you feel strongly repulsed by something, investigate why. You might find that your aversion is a leftover habit you no longer need. (If this idea intrigues you, we talk more about it in chapter 19.)

17

FEAR OF THE UNKNOWN

Abhinivesha is the fifth klesha, and it's often translated as fear of death or clinging to life. Abhinivesha is an extension of asmita and dvesha; it is an obstacle caused by our ceaseless ego gripping. When we teach this philosophical concept, we often share a funny clip from the now-defunct show *The Colbert Report*, in which Stephen Colbert discusses a study that showed people were happier consuming media when they knew the ending of the story. Extrapolating from this, he suggested that he could provide joy by offering the biggest spoiler of them all: You die.

This particular take brings humor to our death-fear, and in our opinion, adding humor to such a complex thing to contemplate—the end of your known existence—is the right call. But the point Colbert was making is that regardless of who you are or what life you live, the same, inevitable end awaits all of us. Even more importantly, if you recognize that death is inevitable and do your best to engage with this knowledge, rather than shy away from it, suffering and fear actually *lessen*. What replaces them is a drive to enjoy the limited days and hours of your existence, celebrating your life and the love you share with others.

Given that knowledge—that our existence has an expiration date, and we have no choice in that matter—it's wild to consider how many people live a life that is completely motivated by fear of this inevitability. Perhaps that's because, at its heart, abhinivesha is fear of the unknown.

Whether you have a faith tradition you practice or you have a humanistic worldview, you likely recognize that it is impossible to understand what awaits after death. (That is why faith is *faith*.) Consider that the unknown generally creates a sense of unease. If you've ever witnessed someone who just walked into a surprise party, you've seen this in action: Even as they begin to realize that there is a joyous occasion afoot, they can't fully grasp what is happening because it was so unexpected. When we can't anticipate what is to come, it creates anxiety.

From an ego perspective, we can't imagine that we, personally, will end. Attachment and aversion show up here, too: Not only are we attached to life, but we are also averse to not knowing and not having an answer. Death is the *end* of life (ours, our parents', our children's, our loved ones'), and it's also the *beginning* of the unknown. For both of those reasons, we might feel resistance to it.

ACTIONS

What do we do in the face of this inevitable fate that awaits all of us? How do we temper our fear of this unknown and not allow abhinivesha to control us? Here are a few practical suggestions.

Lean into the unease of not knowing. Notice if you have a well-practiced desire to know, plan, or be in control. Investigate that. Explore it. Does being in control allow you to feel safe? Are there moments that you can try experiencing a sense of safety or, if not quite that, joyous exhilaration, in *not* knowing? In practice, this might look like resisting the urge to plan every moment of a vacation or handing the reins of an important day off to a loved one to fully oversee. Notice when you feel unease about the unknown, whether that is trying a new food or hiking a less-used trail. Notice the fear at the heart of the unease. Notice, too, when that fear is unfounded (the food was delicious!) and when it was founded (that trail was extremely advanced) and notice that in either case, things probably turned out more or less OK.

See the joy in death. Funerals are often incredibly poignant, full of loving tributes and happy memories and gratitude that the loved one, now gone, was a part of our lives. It's not an exaggeration to say that funerals can be occasions of joy and richness. Sometimes death brings us closer to others. Often, it helps us better understand ourselves. Occasionally, the death of a loved one can be a catalyst for deep healing. The fact that life has an endpoint enriches it deeply.

Make death a part of your meditations. *Memento mori*; remember that you must die. Instead of turning away from death, follow the lead of artists through the centuries and include a reminder of it in your everyday life. The fly or the skull in a still-life painting is there to remind us of the inevitability of decay and death. So how about trying this as a mantra: "None of this matters, and we all die." You can interpret this in two markedly different ways: It can have a tone of futility, or a tone of celebration and reverence. We suggest the latter. After all, if none of this inherently matters, that means you alone get to create your own meaning! Allow this stark and honest assessment of reality to motivate you to be fully present. If none of this matters, then it is up to *you* to determine what matters. If we all die, then it means *you* get to determine what to do with your time until the end. Perhaps you will still feel a lingering fear of the unknown. But consider that there is also great freedom in what we do know as fact: *None of this really matters, and we all die.*

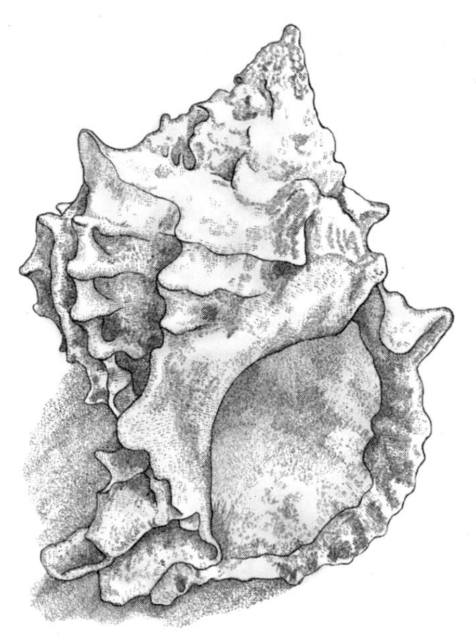

18
STUCKNESS

Habits are critical for your efficient day-to-day operation. Imagine having to design your morning routine from scratch every day! You'd use a full day's worth of mental energy before your coffee was even ready. Instead, you've developed a pattern that might involve a chain of sequential actions: get up, use the bathroom, start the coffee, let the dog out, feed the cat, prepare some breakfast, brush your teeth, and so on. We can use these sort of preexisting action chains for "habit stacking," which is an approach to building healthy habits by adding them on to your existing routine. For example, while the coffee brews or while the dog is in the yard, you could add on twenty bodyweight squats, or ten minutes of meditation, or three rounds of box breathing.

Imagine a grassy field or a pristine forest, free of trails. To get across the field or through the forest, you must forge a new path: This is trail-blazing, literally. Once that initial effort has been expended, every consecutive trip along the same path becomes easier. The grass is tamped down; the underbrush is cleared. It takes less physical and less mental energy to follow this new trail you've laid. You can get where you're going faster, with less effort. Habits can create a similar groove. They are pathways you've set for yourself to follow in the future.

Still, if you keep using this trail and never take another path, what was initially helpful can become harmful. You may wear the grass away, exposing bare earth that's so trodden down that nothing can grow. Or, in the forest, continued usage of a trail can convert it from a clear pathway to a muddy, rocky, perilous mess.

Think back to the roots of a habit: Maybe, as Sage did, you started running as a means of stress release. It took a lot of effort at first, but you quickly saw a big return on that investment: You feel fitter and more centered, and you're getting faster. But at some point the habit tips from a groove to a rut; you hit diminishing returns. What was at first a way to be calm may become a source of obsession, enticing you to make unwise choices to hit a weekly mileage target, or to ignore your body's signs of injury because there's a race on your calendar that you absolutely *must* run. (You can swap "practicing yoga asana" for "running" if you like, as it's a similar trajectory when you get obsessive about your exercise—or any other initially helpful habit.)

Or think of another habit people develop to relieve stress: having a drink at the end of the day. It helps you feel mellow; it makes it easier to unwind, to chat with friends, or to make new ones. But this initially helpful habit can become a rut quickly, and you might find yourself reaching for the bottle more than you ever intended, in ways that are decidedly *not* healthy.

The trick is to leverage the positive effects of habits—getting into a groove—without letting them become mindless ruts. The Sanskrit word for these habits is *samskara*, sometimes translated as thought-patterns or mental impressions. (It's not the same word as *samsara*, the wheel of life.) When you find yourself feeling stuck in habits or patterns that you know don't ultimately serve you in any good way, you're in a rut, not a groove, and it's time to forge a new trail.

ACTIONS

Here are some practical suggestions.

Pause. When you find yourself in a rut, the first step to get out of it is to do nothing—that is, *stop digging*. Drop the actions that are causing you suffering. If you're running yourself into injury, for example, the first thing to do is to decrease your mileage, maybe even all the way down to zero. When you're mindlessly scrolling on your phone, or closing apps only to immediately reopen them, stop digging: Put the phone down, or better, turn it off.

Switch it up. Because your mind will dislike the void created by stopping a bad habit, it can be helpful to replace the unproductive habit with a new one. That's why smokers switch to gum when they quit. It's still a habit (even, arguably, a rut), but it's a good step in moving away from the most harmful version of that habit. This is a similar approach to breaking cravings by using a benign placeholder, which we suggested in chapter 16. Going for a walk is almost always a great way to break out of your rut. So is getting on your yoga mat, calling a dear friend, or simply going outside to sit in the sunshine. The key is to make a small change. That can be as simple as turning on music or adjusting your seating. Make a shift of some sort.

Rewrite your thoughts. The next step for changing action, for changing the narrative, or for changing in general is to notice how *your thoughts* are a big part of what's keeping you stuck. If you think, "I'm at my happiest when I can run daily," then that thought is true. But as we explored in chapter 10, the teaching of cognitive reappraisal (*pratipaksha bhavana*) prompts us to imagine things from a different perspective or try on an opposite thought. "I'm at my happiest when I can run daily" becomes "I'm at my happiest when I can move my body" or even "I get to decide my happiness, no matter what movement I can do." In time, the new mental trail will be forged and the stuckness will start to resolve.

19
HIDDEN COMPULSIONS

Vasanas are similar to samskaras. If we view samskaras as the ruts of stuck habits, then vasanas are the compulsions behind these habits. These compulsions—usually hidden from our conscious mind—are the seeds of a great deal of suffering. When you act from an unconscious place, it's unlikely that you're taking much of the present moment into account. We define *vasana* as "impression" or "tendency," but you might imagine it as the trace of past events that still causes present action. This isn't always a bad thing. You can think of vasana like a lingering scent: It's a delight to walk into a house where cookies were recently baked! But it's less delightful to walk into a well-used public restroom. In both cases, the past aroma is lingering and creating the fragrance of the present.

We might also compare the concept of vasana to the way machine learning works. With this type of technology, computer systems learn to identify patterns or make predictions based on data. Sometimes these systems "learn" from interactions with people asking questions, offering feedback, and seeking clarification. You're the same. Consider all of your life experiences: every interaction with another person, every childhood event, every relationship and friendship, every place you've lived or visited. This has all become part of your mental operating system, part of the software code that defines how you see the world and how you respond to it. Unless you spend time uncovering how your experiences have created who you are now, you'll be limited to only the code that's been written.

There's a lot of talk in modern self-help culture about the "shadow self," and vasanas are a good example of that. Your shadow self is the part of yourself that you repress or you don't acknowledge. It may be something you're lightly aware of, but it brings you shame or discomfort, so you don't engage with it often. To know what's there, why it's there, and what wisdom it's offering you, you have to get to know all of the parts of yourself, even the parts that you don't like or want. You have to understand the tendencies and compulsions behind your behavior.

ACTIONS

Moving through vasanas involves self-reflection.

Journal. You know when it's time for a mental software update or repatterning. For example, we bet you are aware of some self-limiting beliefs from your childhood that you're hanging on to. Write about those. Or, if you're not sure what events from your past are the ghosts of your present, work backward: Write about what you see as the most important events or relationships of your life and unpack what you learned from those events. You'll find that many of your current tendencies for self-protection, for instance, arise from something that is no longer a threat to you.

Reflect with others. Therapy helps you overwrite your outdated software code with something more useful. You may know that you're limited by your own history, but knowing that is only the start. As with samskara, you can't get out of the rutted trail without finding another trail to walk on. With vasana, how can you better understand the things that have happened in your life so that your history doesn't leave such a strong imprint on the present? You have to know your past, know your tendencies in the now, and find new ways to be in and view the world that challenge those tendencies—especially when they are the cause of suffering.

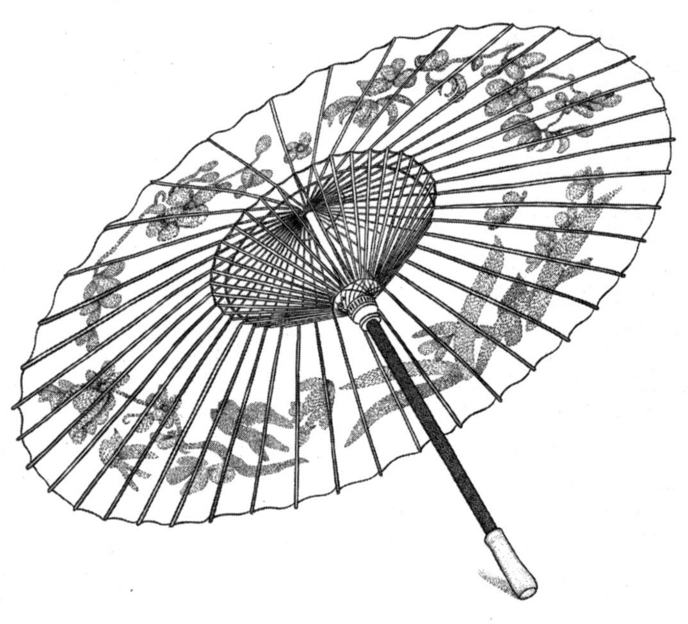

20

THE ILLUSION OF SEPARATENESS

We've talked already about how a sense of separateness is at the heart of all pain. We call this imagined division *maya*. Maya is the illusion of separateness from divinity that causes us to cling to the material world and try to find solvency there. Because of maya, you overidentify with ego or you take things much more seriously than you need to.

There's a Hafiz poem, translated by Daniel Ladinsky as "Tripping Over Joy," that describes a chess game taking place between a mystic and the Divine. In the poem, the mystic is uproariously laughing over the amazing moves by God's hand; they know that it's all a game. In contrast, an uninitiated human (who sees God as separate from themself) may think they are playing a very serious game, one that they have a real chance of winning. The mystic surrenders to all the plays in the game; the skeptic spends far too much time plotting moves that do not matter.[1]

That's maya. If you believe that your current reality is the only reality or is somehow separate from everything else, then you are deluded into believing that your small part *is* the whole. On the other hand, when you are able to see yourself as part of a larger system, as part of everything—every breathing being, every star in the cosmos, every grain of sand on the beaches—then the veil of maya is lifted, and you can see reality without the illusion of separateness. It's in this moment that you recognize that you're in divinity and you yourself are divine—along with everything else in existence.

ACTIONS

Immerse yourself in the mystical. There's an open movement toward exploring hallucinogenic substances as an opportunity to immerse yourself in the divine. And while we're not opposed to immersion in the mystical in this form, you can also have similar experiences that don't make use of these substances. Consider the collective effervescence at a concert. The euphoria of synchronous singing and dancing is a mystical experience that can remind you that you are not a fully unique expression of existence. In these moments, the veil is lifted and you can see how you are one with others. Seek out these mystical experiences, whether they are in the form of therapeutic retreat, ecstatic concert-going, or Sunday-morning hymn singing.

See the mystical in everyday life. Conversely, you don't need a big event to lift the veil. Notice the ways you are like others. See a stranger wearing a shirt you also own as evidence that we are all beings of the divine, come to play on this earth together. Notice how other parents love their children (or four-legged children) the way you love yours. Take note, too, of when you are aware of yourself as *very different* from another person. See that difference as an example not of division but of how the divine takes many forms—some of which you may never understand in this lifetime.

21

THE ILLUSION OF TIME

In the third chapter of the Yoga Sutras, yogic powers (*siddhis*) are revealed. Whether or not these powers exist in the literal sense is up for debate. (Neither of us have ever levitated, but let us know if you have!) In sutra 3.16, recognizing that time is an illusion is presented as a sort of superpower. Sometimes the translation of this sutra suggests something like, "Deep meditation will allow you to access both past lives and premonitions of future happenings." Put like that, it certainly sounds like a magic power—although not one we're really sure we would want.

But another way to understand this sutra is to see it as a reminder that time is an illusion. You've already experienced this: Consider a time when you were stuck waiting in a line, and every five minutes that passed felt more like an hour. Next, reflect on a time when you were excited about an upcoming event. When it finally arrived, time seemed to go faster than normal. Maybe that week in Paris flew by! You know that time is an illusion, even if it is one that we have all colluded in. In fact, that's why it is sometimes called the "grand illusion"; we all look at the same clock and allow the numbers to mean the same thing. We collectively agree on weekends and holidays. We have a shared cultural experience regarding what happens at certain times of day, what happens at certain ages, what happens in certain grades in school.

Time as we're considering it here, though, is not completely about the hours in a day or the days in a week. Instead, it's about your *perception* of the relationship between your past, present, and future. These three states of being—what you were, what you are, and what you will be—are reflected in the cyclical nature of all life: You were born, you now exist, and you will die.

If your perception of time is that it is passing quickly or not in the way that you hoped it would, you will move in the world with a scarcity mentality—fearful of the impending end, concerned about what legacy you will leave, and feeling as though you will never achieve enough. You might glorify the feeling of being busy, believing on some level that your industriousness will buy you more time. Your busy days can create an illusion of fullness that allows you to be distracted from time ticking on.

Similarly, if you stay rooted in the past, holding on to beliefs, memories, and "how things used to be," you're likely to view the present through a lens of fear or dislike. After all, it's hard for the reality of the present to compete with a magical reminiscence of the past. Looking at the past, you may forget discomforts or hardships that were part of it; it's more difficult to ignore bothers and pains happening in the immediate *now*.

The practice of yoga can help you approach the passage of time not with a sense of scarcity or loss but rather a sense that you are part of an ongoing cycle of creation, preservation, and destruction. In relation to your physical body, you may see past, present, and future as three distinct times. But stepping back a little can allow you to see time as a compressed, single thing and a continuous, ongoing cycle. Where you are in that cycle matters less when you recognize that it is never-ending, never-ceasing.

We collude in the illusion of time because we need it to create a shared reality from which we can functionally operate. But the past, present, and future are all parts of the same whole.

ACTIONS

Lose time. Clocks and time are a ubiquitous part of our lives. We bet that right now, as you're reading this, you have access to the exact time—either on your wrist, on your e-reader, on a nearby clock, or on your phone. When do you ever get to wander the world with no worries about time? Find opportunities to lose time. The next time you take a hike, put your phone away and vow not to check it until you're back at your car. (Sage convinced her editor at *Runner's World* to run the Big Sur International Marathon with her watch-free, and they still came in together, just under their goal time!) Or take on an event or activity without letting a certain time dictate its end. Go to the beach and leave only when you're ready to go, not because you have some preconceived notion of when you should arrive back home. Allow yourself to exist in moments without concern for what was before or what will be after.

Take control over your time. Not every moment of the day should be spent on industriousness, nor should every moment of the day be spent on leisure. But you need to spend time on both. (In equal amounts, we would argue, but your bank account may not agree.) Make it a habit to schedule both work and leisure. Commit to chunks of time to read, go for a walk, or better yet, do nothing. Put it on your calendar in your favorite color. When the "do nothing" time arrives, resist the urge to scroll your phone. Instead, give yourself license to do something organizational, creative, or relaxing. Ironically, by scheduling this free time for yourself, you'll have more of a chance to immerse yourself in the now.

22

SUFFERING IS INEVITABLE

The Yoga Sutras tell us that suffering (*dukha*) that has not yet arisen may be avoided. We cannot avoid all suffering, nor should we. Suffering is an innate part of life, and it is an experience that connects us all in our shared humanity. But we *can* minimize our role in creating or adding to our own future suffering (and the suffering of others). Suffering often happens when we jump out of the present moment and begin anxiously fretting about something that may or may not ever come to pass. Our anxiety is prone to overestimating how bad things will be and underestimating our ability to handle whatever comes to pass—and this leads to unneeded suffering.

The Buddha described this situation as the "two arrows." The first arrow brings the suffering that's inevitable in the course of a life. It's neutral, impersonal, unavoidable. As we already noted, to exist is to experience some suffering. The *second* arrow, though, is the one we shoot at ourselves by assigning aversion or other negative reactions to the suffering. This second arrow is avoidable. The act of avoiding the suffering that could be coming our way is to refrain from shooting that second, self-inflicted arrow.

Those who have committed to endurance sports know that if you want to perform well, some suffering is inevitable. If you want to see what you're made of—how long or how fast you can go—you must confront this edge. In fact, changing your relationship to suffering is probably much of what impels you to sign up for a marathon, a triathlon, or a through-hike. Those of us who seek these experiences want to leverage the inevitability of suffering and use it as a forge for our souls—to go into the fire and use it to burn away the nonessential parts of our being. We see the training and the race as a laboratory where we conduct research on the nature and meaning of our existence. In this way, we court and confront suffering intentionally to build our comfort with it, so that when it arises in the course of life, we don't increase it by resisting it.

Another way to think of this is to recognize moments when unfounded fear creates more suffering than what you're actually afraid of. Alexandra hated shots and needles as a child. There was no real reason for this; they didn't really hurt, they were over quickly, and they were infrequent in her relatively healthy childhood. The suffering of a momentary vaccine was far overshadowed by the suffering caused by the irrational fear that Alexandra felt at the prospect of getting a shot. That sort of unnecessary suffering is exactly what we want to (and can) avoid.

The word for this avoidable suffering, *duhka*, literally means "bad axle space," referring to the cutout at the center of a wheel that allows it to turn smoothly. When this axle hole is out of alignment—when it's off-center or cut unevenly—it takes more effort for the wheel to spin. The ride is more bumpy. The wheel itself wears down sooner. Similarly, dukha stems from being out of alignment—with your values, with reality, and with the truth of the present moment. You come back into alignment by ceasing resistance to the now.

ACTIONS

Cold plunge. Though it's quite trendy right now—and though the science on its effectiveness as a recovery modality is murky—a cold plunge can help change your relationship with suffering.[1] It elicits a strong reaction that you might initially interpret as pain or suffering, but on deeper investigation and exploration this feeling may resolve into mere discomfort or strong sensation. A few minutes in an ice bath or a chilly body of water can help you discern between uncomfortable sensation and actual suffering. And, like running a marathon, it feels so good when it's over!

Reflect on anticipation versus reality. Our anxiety—one of those "second arrows"—tells us that things are going to be worse than they actually are and that we are going to be less capable of handling things than we actually are. This overestimation of circumstance and underestimation of our resilience are both manifestations of *maya*, illusion, which we explored in chapter 20.

After a situation that you've fretted about—a job interview, a surgery, an uncomfortable conversation—take some time to reflect on what you feared would happen versus what actually did happen, and on what you thought you couldn't handle versus what you actually could. Consider thoughtfully whether your fretting made things better or worse. If you are self-aware enough, you might even write down beforehand what your mind-fluctuations are telling you the worst-case scenario could be. Putting this in writing might show you that you're exaggerating. Then afterward, compare what you feared with what happened. This literal reality check strengthens your mindfulness of what is truly real, and it keeps you from piercing yourself with that second arrow and piling on avoidable suffering.

PART IV

INTEGRATE YOUR WHOLE SELF:
MODELS OF BEING AND HOW TO HARMONIZE THEM

We've seen that yoga offers a take on both the positive and negative elements of human experience. In this part of the book, we'll explore five different models of our being—the koshas, the chakras, the doshas, the vayus, and the gunas—and ways to harmonize them, so that we can be fully integrated on an energetic and spiritual level.

There is no need to assign positive or negative attributes to parts of any of these models; instead, we use them as a way into ourselves. We also don't have to integrate all of the models. Maybe the doshas make more sense to you than the chakras. Great! Learn more about the doshas and use them to better understand yourself. Remember the joy of the yogic system of spirituality: It's not dogmatic. There is nothing here you need to believe or not believe. Take from it what most resonates for you. Perhaps the best way to conceive of these models, then, is to imagine them as tools; they are just metaphors that give you more options for understanding who you are in the world.

As you read, you'll notice that many of these models map onto each other; that isn't by accident. Our models here break down into groups of odd numbers: there are seven chakras; five koshas and five vayus; and three doshas and three gunas. In part V, we'll move on to pairs of energies that balance with each other to keep the integration of your being going.

Most of these models point to what's called the energetic body or subtle body, including the vayus, the chakras, and the koshas. While the concept of the subtle body is pervasive in our experience of the world, we don't have great words for it. In modern parlance, we might say something like "aura" or "vibes" when referring to the energies in us and around us. There are sometimes correlations between the subtle body and the physical body, but not always. The subtle body is not something that needs to be scientifically proven or disproven. Subtle-body models are intuitive ways to feel the world, and they can be quite revelatory on your personal path to self-discovery and awakening.

23

INTEGRATING THE LAYERS OF YOUR SELF: *THE KOSHAS*

The koshas offer us a complete model for the subtle body by describing the layers of your being from the outside in, from the gross and external to the subtle and internal. These layers are like a set of nested lampshades filtering the divine light within you, so that it presents a little differently at every concentric ring.

If you've ever enjoyed yoga nidra, a form of guided relaxation, you likely were taken on a journey through the koshas, from the outer layer to the inner and back out again. That's part of why yoga nidra is so deeply calming: It resonates within you on an intangible, subtle level. But you don't have to practice yoga nidra to experience awareness of the koshas; you can bring this into your everyday life, too.

Annamaya Kosha (The Physical Sheath): When you identify with your body, this is the part you're connecting to. Annamaya kosha is both the densest and the most superficial layer of yourself. This is the part of you that is easiest to see, so it can also too easily become the part that you think of as the *you* you, when instead there are so many more layers to you. Getting to know the kosha model is one way to remember that there's way more to you than annamaya kosha, the layer that meets the eye.

That's not to say that the physical sheath isn't deeply important! Of course it is. Whether you're in pain or comfortable, whether you're healthy or injured, whether you're feeling good about your appearance or not—all of that can affect you on a spiritual and emotional level. That's why caring for your appearance is not always vanity, nor is a desire to build a strong physical body necessarily rooted in self-obsession. Without health or vitality or a certain level of comfort with your appearance, you may feel deeply stuck in this koshic layer, unable to focus on anything but the physical sheath of your blood and bones. Caretaking of this sheath is important, mostly so you are not distracted by it in a way that means you are unable to see the deeper layers of your subtle body.

Pranamaya Kosha (The Breath Body): Take a full breath in. You feel that in your physical body, but you feel it somewhere else, too. (Now let the breath go, if you haven't yet!) It's hard to pin down what you're feeling, exactly, but it's a reminder that there is a life force that animates your physical body. Were you to cease breathing, your outermost layer would remain, but it would be static, inanimate. Just as *prana* means both "breath" and "life force," your pranamaya kosha is both your breath body and the energetic layer that gives you life.

Manomaya Kosha (The Thinking and Feeling Sheath): When you're reminded not to identify with your thoughts or feelings, this is what you should imagine. Your thoughts and feelings are you, but they're not the complete picture of who you are. Manomaya kosha is the layer of you that—despite being less tangible than body or breath—speaks the loudest. It has all the thoughts, all the moods, all the wants and needs. That's why it's so very helpful to notice that this is but *one* layer, one part of you—there's lots more within and without.

Vijnanamaya Kosha (The Intuitive Layer): Beneath the loudest layer is the still, small voice within that already knows the truth and whispers its wisdom. It's your gut knowledge, the deep truth you hold. Sometimes this wisdom rushes out in a gush, and you're unable to ignore the sparkling brilliance of the truth it suddenly reveals. (Consider moments that have felt revelatory, when an idea or the right answer to some life puzzle has just *come* to you.) Sometimes, though, the wisdom of your intuition is quieter and harder to hear, and you have to find the space, time, and energy to tune into it, trust it, and abide by what it tells you. This is why being healthy in your physical body, attuned to your energetic body, and aware of your thoughts and feelings—and knowing that they are each only one part of the whole— matters so much. It reduces the static that can scramble the signal between your intuitive body and your conscious awareness.

Anandamaya Kosha (The Bliss Body): Your true nature is the radiant lightbulb that the lampshades of the other layers have been covering. So many concepts in yoga interweave with one another, and this is an excellent example of that. Your anandamaya kosha might also be defined as the part of you that experiences samadhi or the layer of you that truly knows you are divine.

ACTIONS

Scan through the layers. Your yoga asana or other movement practices are a good setting for this scan, as they tune you in first to your body and then to your breath—so you are already two layers deep. At the start of your practice, you might notice the noise of manomaya kosha and see if there is anything to attend to there. As your practice unfolds—perhaps in the quiet moments of shapes like child's pose—you can pause to hear any messages of wisdom unfurling from vijnanamaya kosha. Finally, as you settle into savasana, notice the bliss. That bliss comes from your exhausted body, but it's far, far more than that. In this stillness, your radiant nature may become more obvious.

Notice which "you" is which layer. On the path toward integrating all the koshas, you might notice which is which. For instance, the "you" that cannot find an outfit that feels right or comfortable on an early Monday morning is most likely your annamaya kosha. The "you" that steps out the door on a bright morning and breathes in as deeply as possible is your pranamaya kosha. The "you" that chatters away or feels mad about something meaningless is undoubtedly your manomaya kosha. And the "you" that knows itself and desires truly is your vijnanamaya kosha. The "you" that laughs easily, that snuggles with your child or your kitty or a good book—that "you" is your anandamaya kosha. When you start to see these layers in your words, actions, desires, laughter, and deep breaths, you get less attached to any one layer. Noticing the voices of these various layers helps you see that they are *all* you, and not one of them is you alone.

Do a yoga nidra practice. Since yoga nidra is typically facilitated as an exercise to move you through these layers, you should absolutely try it. You can probably find a yoga nidra offering at your favorite studio. If not, you can do this at home, following along to a recorded version. (Sage has one on offer at www.sagerountree .com/yogaoffthemat.)

24

THE HIERARCHY OF NEEDS: *THE CHAKRAS*

The idea that there are energetic channels or lines running through the body comes from some of the most ancient yoga. We see evidence of this in the Upanishads, where these energetic channels are called *nadis*. Some tantric texts report that there are as many as 72,000 nadis. Nadis help move pranic energy around and through the body; they are roughly analogous to the meridians in Traditional Chinese Medicine. When energy is flowing freely through these channels, you feel good—you're mentally, physically, and spiritually well. When energy gets stuck or caught up somewhere, you don't feel so good.

Ida and *pingala* are the main left and right energetic channels, respectively, and *sushumna nadi* is the central one; ida and pingala spiral concentrically around sushumna, and in the places where they cross, you'll find a *chakra*: an energetic center in the body. Sushumna is also the channel through which *kundalini*—the higher spiritual consciousness—rises up from its origin at the *muladhara chakra* (at the base of the spine) to *sahasrara chakra* (at the crown of the head). In subtle-body terms, the sushumna nadi is the path to enlightenment. That's one reason we devote time and attention to awareness of the energy in the body; you want to keep the way to liberation free of obstacles.

The idea of chakras doesn't show up in yogic texts until the rise of tantra—some time after the concept of the nadis was developed. There is some disagreement about the number of chakras: Some tantric schools suggest that there are five chakras, while others identify the seven we've come to know in our Western yoga. Some purport that there are many more chakras than that.[1] Rather than take this as evidence that there is no "true" chakra system, remember that the chakras—like all the subtle-body systems we elucidate in this book and that are elaborated on in other yogic texts—are opportunities for self-discovery. They are not tangible, absolute truths. (It's pretty rare that any teaching of yoga claims to be *the* absolute truth, and we'd encourage you to be skeptical if you encounter a yoga teacher who suggests this.)

The rainbow colors we often associate with the chakras were applied even more recently. They may have first shown up in the 1927 book *The Chakras* by C. W. Leadbeater.[2] Some time after this, the colors were codified and standardized in popular books like Anodea Judith's *Eastern Body, Western Mind.*[3] The rainbow colors of the chakras can help you visualize these energy centers, which is why we use them here. Like many other models in the yoga system, the chakras are a palimpsest: There's a deep truth at play here, but it is one that has been interpreted by many different thinkers and cultures through the years. Take the parts that work for you. If they help you feel more self-aware and present, or if they make you kinder to everyone you come into contact with, they are useful.

Muladhara is the root chakra (red). Its physical location is at the bottom of your torso, at the base of your spine. This chakra governs safety, stability, and self-preservation. Muladhara chakra is concerned with basic needs like survival, shelter, connection, and family bonding. This chakra may need attention when life presents big changes or when there is a substantial amount of fear you're working through. When muladhara is in balance, you may feel a sense of trust in the flow of life; you feel cared for and in harmony with the world around you. Consider the moments in which you have most been aware of muladhara—maybe you sensed its imbalance in a moment when you felt physically unsafe or you were injured. Or maybe you've experienced energy moving through this chakra while visiting your childhood home or spending time with a beloved grandparent.

Svadhisthana is the sacral chakra (orange). Its physical location is below your belly button, at the site of your reproductive organs. This chakra governs emotions, creativity, sensuality, and sexuality. This chakra may need attention if you feel vulnerable or dissatisfied in an important relationship. When svadhisthana chakra is out of balance, you may feel that you can't trust others. When it is in balance, though, svadhisthana chakra allows you to take creative risks and enjoy the sweet moments in life. When have you seen or felt svadhisthana most active and free-flowing? You might remember a time when you were in a creative streak with an artistic project, writing or painting away. Or you may connect this chakra to the feeling of awakening that begins at the start of a new relationship.

Manipura is the solar-plexus chakra (yellow). Its physical location is at your navel. This chakra governs self-esteem and personal power; it connects to how you get your needs met. (Some Chinese movement practices like tai chi and qigong have a similar concept called the *dantian*, situated a little lower than the navel.) An imbalance in this chakra may leave you feeling unworthy or criticized. When manipura is in balance and energy is flowing freely, you'll feel a strong sense of inner peace and wholeness. You've noticed manipura chakra when you've felt most powerful: for example, when you nail the presentation at work or cross the finish line in record time. When you feel proud of yourself—not in an egocentric way, but with regard to who you are deeply as a person and the way you walk in the world—then you have felt manipura chakra moving and flowing freely.

Anahata is the heart chakra (green). Its physical location is your heart space. This chakra largely governs relationships. Anahata chakra concerns itself with forgiveness, trust, empathy, and generosity. It's this chakra that helps you be aware of others' needs. Anahata out of balance might look like holding on to grief or anger; a lack of sympathy for others; and a lack of close, loving relationships. In balance, anahata shows up as compassion for others. In moments when you have been moved deeply by others, when you feel your humanity rise to meet the humanity of others, anahata chakra is awakening. When you feel like you can love freely with no withholding—when you walked down the aisle or held your child for the first time—anahata chakra governs those moments.

Vishuddha is the throat chakra (blue). It is located at the base of the throat. This chakra governs communication in all forms. Vishuddha chakra concerns itself with inner voice, speaking your truth, and personal authority. When this chakra needs attention, it may show up as a sense that you can't say what you mean or can't communicate effectively—or even that you can't stop talking! Vishuddha chakra gets out of balance if you don't feel heard, if you're not listening to your inner voice, or if you don't feel free to speak your personal truth. When vishuddha is in balance, you have strong communication skills and are able to stand firmly in your truth without hiding. Can you remember a moment in which you shared something with another person that felt really hard? Maybe you told someone your true feelings about them or asked for something you needed. In those moments, your vishuddha chakra center was uninhibited.

Ajna is the third-eye chakra (indigo). It is located in the center of your forehead, between and slightly above your eyes. This chakra governs integrity, thought, and logic. Ajna empowers your sense of perceptions and beliefs. Out of balance, ajna chakra shows up as a lack of personal purpose or a sense of deep confusion. In balance, it feels like you are guided by a clear sense of intuition and knowing what you believe to be true. When you've felt a sense of being on the right side of history, when you've known deep truth, goodness, and the right course of action—that is ajna chakra unfettered.

Sahasrara is the crown chakra (violet). This chakra is located at the very top of your head—your crown. Sahasrara chakra governs your sense of awe and connection to the divine. Its crucial aspects include faith, devotion, and insight. A crown chakra that is out of balance may feel like loneliness, isolation, and a sense of disconnection from others and from the divine. In balance, free-flowing sahasrara reveals a feeling of unity, a rejection of ego, and a recognition that self is an extension of Self.

Here's a good way to approach the seven chakras. As you familiarize yourself with these seven energetic centers of the body, which one calls to you the most? Which do you immediately recognize as a place that needs work? This may be the best chakra to begin working with.

If you're familiar with Abraham Maslow's hierarchy of needs, you'll notice its resonance with the chakras. This concept is usually depicted as a pyramid, the base of which represents our most basic needs of physical safety and health; as we move up the pyramid, successive layers represent other needs such as "belonging" and "self-esteem," and culminating in self-actualization. As you investigate the chakras and how they can help you know yourself, if you don't feel called to start at any particular one of them, another approach might be to similarly move up them one by one, from the bottom to the top.

ACTIONS

Chakra sound clearing. This practice involves taking a restful shape—like something you'd practice in a restorative yoga class or a well-supported sitting position—and working your way through the chakras while chanting their "seed sounds," or bija mantras:

- Root chakra: *lam*

- Sacral chakra: *vam*

- Solar-plexus chakra: *ram*

- Heart chakra: *yam*

- Throat chakra: *ham*

- Third-eye chakra: *om*

- Crown chakra: silence

You'll find videos of this online, if you need to see an example of what sound clearing looks (and sounds) like. At its core, it's very simple. Try this practice in savasana with cushy props, or lie on your bed with a pillow under your head and, if you like, another under your knees.

Bring your attention to your root chakra. Chant, either aloud or silently, *lam lam lam lam lam*. (You can pronounce the *a* in each of these mantras more like a *u*, so this sounds almost like *lump* without the *p*.) Keep going until you feel like moving on—but before you do, pause and feel the vibrations, keeping your attention on your root chakra. Then move up the chain.

If you like, you can layer on some color meditation, visualizing each chakra's color before moving to the next one.

Investigate the chakras. Approach the chakras with a sense of curiosity about what you can learn about yourself. You might journal or meditate on questions that help you connect to how free-flowing or stagnant each chakra is. Use this to guide future practices, like deeper meditation, targeted therapy sessions, or yoga asanas that emphasize the body parts closest to where the target chakra resides.

- Muladhara: When do I feel most safe? What practices bring about my sense of resiliency and constancy? What makes me feel most unsafe? Are there times in my life that I felt afraid? Is there more work I need to do so I can know I am OK now?

- Svadhisthana: When I sit with the idea of being "creative," does resistance or discomfort come up? Do I see myself as a creative person? When I feel my most free and open, what's happening around me? Who am I with and what am I doing?

- Manipura: What makes me feel my most confident and powerful? Are there certain people or situations that make me feel the opposite of that? Can I limit my time in those places?

- Anahata: Who freely gets my love? Why do I find loving them to be an easy task? When am I most aware of my capacity for compassion? What exhausts my compassion?

- Vishuddha: Are there places in my life where I am not being my full self or speaking my truth? What would happen if I were to be completely honest in these places? Do I have something I need to say? Are there words that feel stuck? Who in my life is easiest for me to communicate with?

- Ajna: Do I listen to my intuition? What does it tell me? Are there times when I ignored my inner knowing? What did it cost me? When am I most aware of my intuition? What circumstances call forth this deeper wisdom in a way that I can hear?

- Sahasrara: When do I feel most connected to the divine or aware of my own divinity? Is it on a yoga mat, in nature, with my family, or kneeling in prayer? Are there certain rituals that especially evoke the divine for me? Do I desire to grow my connection to spirituality? What would that look like in my life?

Create associations. As you investigate the chakras and discover which one or two you want to dive into more deeply, create associations throughout your life that bring these chakras to the forefront of your mind. For instance, if you want to do more work around the heart chakra, start your meditation practice with your hands stacked over your heart. Find heart-shaped totems to place on your altar, in your car, or next to your bed. Since green is associated with this chakra, bring more green into your wardrobe, especially the clothes you wear for yoga practice. When a teacher asks you to set your intention before a yoga practice, let your intention be related to your chakra-healing work.

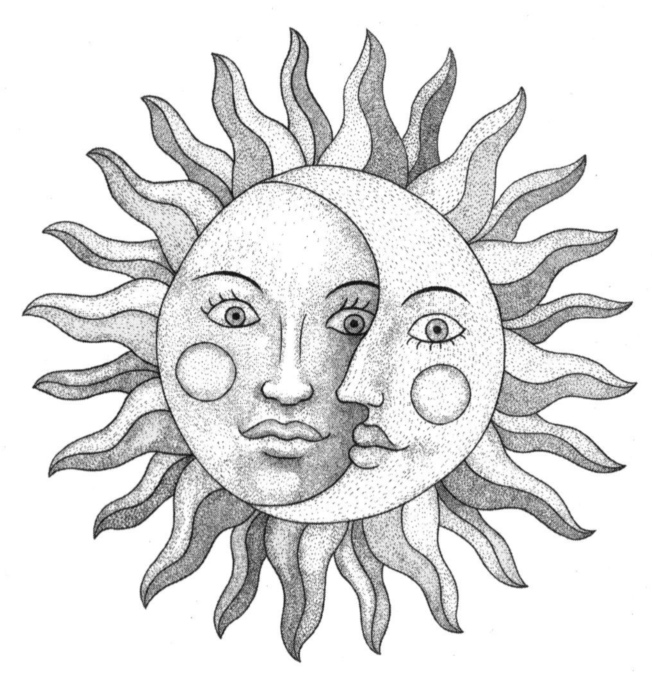

25

LOCKS IN A CANAL: *THE BANDHAS*

You may have encountered the bandhas in the context of a yoga class, where three main bandhas are engaged: *mula bandha*, the root lock; *uddiyana bandha*, the belly lock; and *jalandhara bandha*, the throat lock. *Maha bandha*, the great lock, is a super combo of all three at one time. If you first heard the term *bandha* in an asana practice, it may have been in the context of the physical body only, but these locks are also another manifestation of the subtle or energetic body.

Physically, the bandhas correspond to three areas of your body. Mula bandha corresponds to the bottom of your core and the muscles of your pelvic floor. Uddiyana bandha corresponds to the top of your core and your diaphragm. It is the dividing line between your vital organs and your visceral organs. And jalandhara bandha serves as the throat seal between your head and your heart. Physical engagement of these areas can provide mechanical stability—think of pelvic-floor engagement in a plank pose or in weightlifting. But the goal here goes beyond the physical; it's to seal in the movement of energy, *prana*, in the body. Thus, the three bandhas also correspond with the first, third, and fifth chakras: your base, your gut, and your voice.

Awareness of these regions can draw your attention to the movement of prana in interesting ways. Think of them less as locks that would secure a door and more as locks in a canal. They can be drawn into place to pool energy on one side, then slowly released to even out the energy and move things along, whether they are moving up or moving down, moving in or moving out. (We'll explore these actions in chapter 27 on the *vayus*).

This raises the question: Why would you want to secure energy in certain places in your body? Think about having a conversation with a difficult person. Before you head into the confrontation, you probably prepare yourself both mentally and physically. You might stand taller, draw your chin up, and lightly engage your core. While you may not think of these small shifts as energetic preparations, they are; you're intuitively drawing your energy in tight, preparing for the interaction.

When you engage the bandhas, you may not always be doing it to conserve energy for a challenging situation. Sometimes bandha engagement can be an exploration in feeling how energy flows and stops in your body, as another opportunity to know more about yourself.

ACTIONS

How does it feel to engage the bandhas? This book is about yoga off the mat, but that does not mean being divorced from the physical body. Engaging the three bandhas requires fairly subtle physical shifts; you can engage mula bandha without anyone around you knowing! Engaging mula bandha is similar to turning on the muscles in your pelvic floor, which you would use to stop the flow of urine while using the bathroom. Uddiyana bandha suggests core engagement, but it is less of a muscular engagement of the torso and more like the creation of a vacuum that results in the abdomen hollowing out. For our purposes, though, it's enough to lightly draw attention to your core space. You can cultivate jalandhara bandha by drawing your chin first out, then down and back, so that it lands close to your chest.

Close your eyes and, one at a time, engage and release each bandha. See if you can notice how it feels, not just physically but also energetically. Does it take a lot of effort? Is there discomfort in any of these moments of engagement, or does it feel like relief? Do any of these small physical movements have a spiritual effect?

Energetically prepare yourself for the world. Now that you know how it feels to engage each bandha, consider how you might use this information to broaden your understanding of how your energetic and physical bodies are integrated. How do you want to energetically prepare yourself for the world? And what does that look like, physically? Maybe it means drawing your shoulders back as you enter a new space, so that you feel more aware and alert. If you have to walk to your car in an empty parking lot, perhaps you curl your fingers into your palms—a physical reminder that you are spiritually prepared to protect yourself. It may also mean relaxing your jaw before you give a presentation or putting a smile on your face when you wait in a line. These actions might manifest in the physical, as the bandhas do, but they arise from a thoughtful use of energy.

26

YOUR INHERENT CONSTITUTION:
THE DOSHAS

Ayurveda is a South Asian approach to finding balance in physical and mental wellness. Ayurveda is called the sister science of yoga, and we can think of it as an ancient medical lens through which to view human health. In Ayurveda, the doshas are a set of three categories that explain your temperament, your constitution, and the type of person you innately are. Once you become familiar with these constitutional types, you begin to view yourself and your relationship to others more clearly. In the doshas, we see our yogic practice meet the Ayurvedic worldview.

Sometimes personality-typing models we use for self-exploration can feel limiting: They only hand you a prediction of who you are, not an explanation of how to *be* who you are. The doshas, on the other hand, can help you expand your understanding of who you are while also giving you key knowledge to help you accept yourself as you are—and how to use that knowledge to be the best version of yourself. Perhaps that's why we like the dosha model; santosha is inherent in it.

The doshas are a reminder that all personality types have strengths and weaknesses, and that all of us are a combination of *all* the types, just in different proportions. The goal here is not to achieve some magical energetic balance between all three doshas. It's instead to enhance the good that's already in you—to be who you are, but in a healthy balance within your dosha. As you read the following descriptions, don't be surprised if you see a little of yourself in each one. (But we bet you'll recognize yourself mostly in one.)

Kapha dosha is a grounded, reflective energy. In balance, it confers steadiness, calm, and intentionality. A person with kapha energy is reliable, deliberate, and dependable. Kapha types are homey, loving, and sensible. They tend to prefer routine over chaos, often striving for harmony over adventure. Kapha dosha embodies the earth and water elements. If you're kapha, you might be drawn to relaxing, calming yoga practices—although you may need to try out some more challenging, fiery ones! Out of balance, kapha slides into stubbornness, inaction, lethargy, habituation, and resistance to change.

Vata dosha is a creative, generative energy. In balance, it moves us to make art, to come up with new ideas, and to express ourselves. Vata types may love new projects, new ideas, and new adventures. Vata energy can be infectious in its enthusiasm. Vata dosha embodies the ether and air elements. If you're vata, you might love creative flow sequences but know that you likely need more seated meditation. Out of balance, vata skews toward anxiety, insecurity, and unreliability.

Pitta dosha is the dosha of fiery action. In balance, pitta dosha moves us to decisiveness, to completion of projects, and to meeting deadlines. Pitta types are leaders who tend to get things done. They take initiative and both plan and carry out plans. Pitta dosha embodies the elements of fire and water. If you're pitta, you might enjoy spicy practices like hot power flow but could use the sweetness and stillness of restorative and yin yoga. Out of balance, pitta can slant toward unchecked anger, power-grabbing, resentment, irritability, and jealousy.

If you enjoy this model, you'll find there are many resources available to help you uncover more about your dosha type and bring it into balance.

ACTIONS

Take a quiz. If you can't already discern which of these doshas rules your temperament, you'll find hundreds of quizzes online. They ask you to look at intangible things, like your natural inclinations, as well as to assess physical attributes, like the color of your fingernails or the quality of your digestion. Maintain a healthy skepticism about some of these questions! Even better, have your close family, friends, or partner take a dosha quiz, too. We bet you'll find that in some of the most important relationships in your life, your dosha serves as a complement to your loved one's type.

Get an Ayurvedic assessment or treatment. Find an Ayurvedic practitioner nearby and have an Ayurvedic consultation or a pulse assessment. Even better, try an Ayurvedic treatment or therapy! Our personal favorite is *abhyanga*, a warm oil massage that involves light, relaxing strokes to bring balance to your specific dosha type. If you can find a practitioner, combine the massage with *shirodhara*, the application of a warm stream of oil to your forehead. Not only is it a way to harmonize your doshas, but it's also often a shortcut directly to your bliss body. Once you know your dosha type, you can use it to further enhance your self-care routine according to your personal needs.

27

THE MOVEMENT OF ENERGY: *THE VAYUS*

The *vayus*—translated literally as winds—describe the movement of energy in your body. It might seem esoteric, but once you recognize their movement, you'll notice it throughout your day, and you'll feel more aware of your subtle body when you do. In the yoga teacher training that we run, we ask our trainees to learn both physical anatomy and energetic anatomy. As part of the latter, we identify how the five vayus are expressed in various yoga poses. But the energy that moves through your body is flowing and present off the mat, too.

The vayus appear in early Vedic yogic texts, but they are only briefly referenced in later texts like the Bhagavad Gita and the Yoga Sutras. A helpful way to picture the vayus is to imagine your movement leaving behind streaks of colored wind: energy made visible. For instance, when you jump, that colored wind continues to rise even when your body lands. When you bend or squat, the energy traces downward along your movement. If you lift your arm, not only does your arm rise, but the air above it shifts too. Imagine that air as colored smoke lifting and spreading above you, carrying the upward action forward. Even something like a cough sends a force that travels up and out, with the energy continuing in that direction. In this way, the vayus can be understood as the directional pathways of prana—the ways energy moves within you, around you, and because of your actions. They aren't just trails behind your movement; the five vayus are the animating impulse of the movement itself.

Prana Vayu: Rising Energy

Sometimes we distinguish between Prana with a capital *P*, meaning life-force energy, and prana with a lowercase *p*, meaning rising energy. This is the energy that rises with your inhale: As the air physically moves in and down to your lungs, the energetic action of inhalation is an upward movement. Prana vayu is present when you lift your arms overhead, when you sit up taller in your office chair, and when you take a deep, full breath.

Apana Vayu: Settling Energy

The complement to prana vayu is a downward-moving, settling energy: apana vayu. This is the action of exhalation. Again, even though air is literally moving up from your lungs and out as you exhale, the energetic action of an exhale is downward. Apana vayu is the energy that draws your heels toward the mat in downward-facing dog; it's the energy of your head resting on a pillow at bedtime. It's grounding energy. Apana vayu also governs acts of physical elimination (using the toilet, for instance).

When you use inhales to lift and exhales to lower while you are moving through your asana practice, you're expressing these vayus, riding their energetic waves.

Samana Vayu: Concentrated Energy

Samana vayu moves in toward the center of your body, concentrating energy there. You can think of it as drawing in toward your navel or your third chakra, manipura. Samana vayu is the energy of core-engaging poses. It is also the energy of growing energetically smaller in a crowded room of people or when an argument (or something cringe-inducing) is happening nearby.

Udana Vayu: Expulsive Energy

Udana vayu is the up-and-out energy of singing and chanting, as well as things like coughing or vomiting. Udana vayu is about pulling something from your gut and putting it into the world. And it's necessary—just like a sneeze can't be suppressed, the energy of udana vayu must be released.

Vyana Vayu: Expansive Energy

Vyana vayu is the energy of radiating in every direction. This energy can be a consequence of tapping into udana vayu: Once you expel your voice, for example, you can attenuate and control its expansion out in the world with vyana vayu. Think about the shapes you make in your yoga practice that channel this energy, such as star pose or half moon pose. Vyana vayu also governs the energy you exude in moments of public speaking or when you "own the room."

ACTIONS

Feel these movements of energy in your body. Set down this book and, either in your chair or from standing, move your arms (and legs, if possible) to tap into the vayus. Lift your arms: That's prana vayu. Let them settle: apana vayu. Come to your tiptoes and then settle your heels back to the floor.

Now raise your palms and turn them away from your center, pressing your arms out wide on the horizontal axis: This is vyana vayu, radiating outward. Flip your palms to face your body and slowly draw your hands to your belly: This is samana vayu, concentrating your awareness at your center. Repeat for several rounds.

Finally, pull this concentrated energy from the center of your body up the midline, toward your head, and then press it forward. Think of it like shooting a free throw in basketball, using the ball of energy you've concentrated at your center. This is udana vayu, expulsive energy.

Then maybe play a little: Wiggle, squirm, rise and fall, and without doing any "official" yoga poses, feel how the vayus flow through your body in movement.

Feel these actions in your breath. Now that you're tapped in to the movement of the vayus, feel these actions in your breath. Start with the rising energy of inhalation and the falling energy of exhalation—prana and apana vayu.

After paying attention to a few rounds of breath on this vertical axis, tune in more fully to the action of expelling air—this is the action of udana vayu. Your exhales don't just settle you down energetically, but they also literally move air up and out of your body. And it's not just air, but more precisely, carbon dioxide; each exhalation is a literal release of what you don't need. This carbon dioxide is then synthesized by plants, which exchange it for more oxygen. This is an ongoing energetic cycle that enables life on this planet—all embodied in a universal breath.

As you consider this universal breath, feel the twin energies of samana vayu, concentration toward your core, and vyana vayu, radiating outward. You can emphasize this by drawing inward from your navel and pelvic floor as you exhale and softening outward as you inhale.

Allow your experience of prana vayu to be both literal and metaphorical. If you imagine prana as both breath and life force, can you feel the movement of your life-force energy as you expand and contract, breathing in and out? Imagine this energy flowing through you and around you in various colors, depending on how it moves. Feeling *and* imagining this energy allow you to truly sense it in a way that noticing the breath alone may not.

Once you are tuned in to these movements, notice how they play out across your day. Are there times of the day or activities that emphasize rising energy, such as getting out of bed in the morning? When do you feel the settling energy of apana vayu, other than retiring in the evening and lying in your bed? Where does your energy draw toward center in samana vayu—preparing to walk into a meeting, for example? When does it move up and out with some force in udana vayu? Perhaps it's when you speak up in that meeting, or when you call out to your children. And where do you feel the radiating energy of vyana vayu during your day? For us, this might be while we are practicing yoga asanas or meditating at the end of our practice.

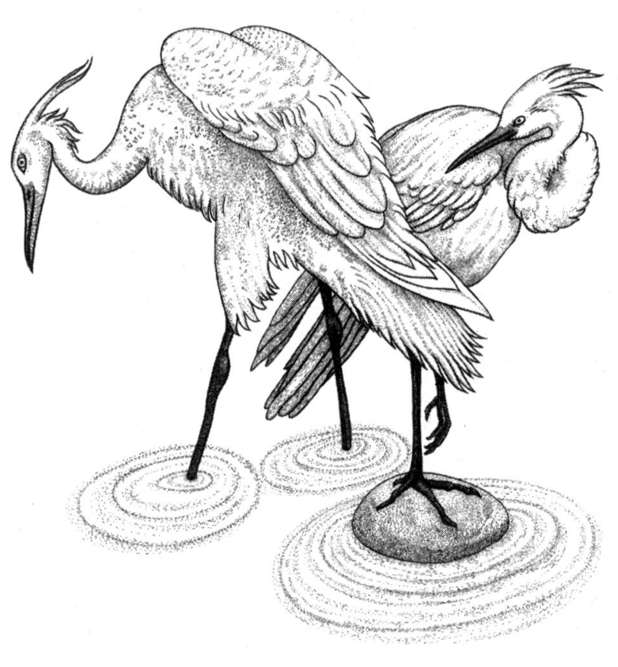

28

LETHARGY, EXCITEMENT, BALANCE: *THE GUNAS*

In yoga cosmology, the *tattvas* are all the elements that make up our existence. Sometimes the tattvas get described as yoga's periodic table of elements, but they aren't necessarily tangible. The tattvas include earth, water, air, fire, and ether, but different schools of yoga philosophy suggest that there are twenty-five to thirty-six tattvas in total. These elements serve as the foundational notes that make up the music of our existence.

The three *gunas*, on the other hand—*tamas, rajas,* and *sattva*—are similarly part of the fabric of our existence, but not as underlying, basic elements. They're something more akin to the flavor of each individual manifestation or aspect of existence. Or, put another way, if the tattvas are individual notes that combine to form music, the gunas are the feelings we get when we listen to that music.

The gunas evoke different characteristics. Tamas is groundedness, lethargy, darkness, and heaviness. Rajas is energy, excitement, brightness, and spontaneity. Sattva is balance, light, rightness, and goodness.

While you probably mostly want to listen to music that evokes beauty, joy, or contentedness, you've probably also desired music that is dark, moody, or sad at different moments in your life. (That's certainly the kind of music we listened to during our early years of relationships and heartbreak!) And we bet when you run on a treadmill or go to a spin class, you prefer music that evokes unlimited energy and a *go-go-go* sense of urgency, with higher beats per minute. In fact, it's easy to see with this example that we need all these types of music—they all have a place in the soundtrack to life.

The gunas are the same: While generally we want the flavor of life to be sattvic, we also need rajas and tamas. Tamas gives us sleep, rest, recovery, and downtime. Tamas is the saddest song you've ever heard, and it's also the kitten napping in the sunbeam. Rajas gives us raucousness, decisive action, and movement. Rajas is running, jumping, playing, and yelling; it's at the heart of getting anything done at all.

Sattva is ease, integrity, and virtue. It's the music that is the most pleasant to listen to; that resolves minor-chord tension into a satisfying major-chord finale; and that evokes mindful and present joy. Sattva is in all things that call you to kindness, to love, and to harmony. And while you need tamas and rajas, most of the time your choices in life should cultivate more sattva. Intuitively, you probably know this. Consider which of these three things makes you feel most truly present and awake to yourself: a Super Bowl party (rajas), a visit to a cemetery (tamas), or a beautiful yoga asana practice with a long savasana (sattva).

ACTIONS

Cultivate sattvic habits. If you imagine the gunas as the background music playing in every moment of your life, how would you create your metaphorical sattvic playlist? Start to identify habits that are the most sattvic. When you wake up in the morning, what's the first thing you do? Do you hit snooze three times in a row, procrastinating getting out of bed? Or do you immediately peruse your to-do list or email, thrusting yourself into work mode? Could you instead wake up and opt for no screen time, spend time outdoors, and allow your mind to awaken and unravel without force or resistance? Sattva begets sattva; if you make choices that bring you to more balance and ease, you will continue to make more choices that do the same. Cultivating sattvic habits might be as simple as noticing how rajas, tamas, and sattva weave through your day and, when possible, choosing the most sattvic path. You might even try charting your habits, writing down which of the gunas they evoke. You need rajas (you have to work and exercise) and tamas (you have to sleep and rest), but in moments when you are not required to move to the melodies of energy or stillness, turn up the volume on the music of goodness and light.

Spend time with sattvic people. Who do you spend time with? What gunas do the people around you evoke? With some reflection, you can probably identify the people that are most tamasic, rajasic, and sattvic in your life. Prioritize being in the company of sattvic people—people who prioritize ethics and kindness, who are less snarky and more authentic, who have a healthy balance of rest and action, and who seem to live with ease. You know whose company is not good for you: the people who make you feel out of sorts or whose choices make you uncomfortable. As much as possible, limit your time with people whose presence cultivates less sattva in you.

Recognizing that you want sattva around you may mean that you end relationships, look for new employment, or spend more or less time with certain family members. Consider that you are drawing these boundaries and making these choices to create more ease and a better, lighter existence for yourself.

When you are unable to opt out of socializing with people whose energy is not the energy you seek for yourself, develop strategies to contain your own sattva in the face of their raja or tamas. That might be as basic as abstaining from drinking around friends who always go overboard or leaving early from a dinner party that creates anxiety. The phrase "protect your peace" applies here. Align yourself with people who are sattvic and reduce your interactions with those who are not.

PART V

KEEP THE
INTEGRATION ALIVE:
PRACTICES OF BALANCE

In the previous chapter, we encouraged you to emphasize the sattvic state in your life and surround yourself with sattvic people. This is because sattva points to balance. The word *balance* often gets associated with the physical practice of yoga, but what does that look like from a philosophical and spiritual standpoint? In this section, we look at what yoga tells us about forces that oppose or complement each other. Investigating practices of balance offers you another perch from which to view your life or the world.

Generally, balance in the spiritual sense is an important aspect of the journey to harmony and freedom: We seek the middle or moderate way of things because it is the most peaceful. Being out of balance or imbalanced (whether physically or spiritually) implies a sense of disharmony, confusion, and ungroundedness. To find a deeper sense of spiritual self, you have to create or uncover balance in yourself.

29

EQUANIMITY AND DISRUPTION

Samatva means equanimity, and it shows up as an important theme in the Bhagavad Gita. In this epic tale, the god Krishna repeatedly implores the warrior Arjuna to be consistent and steady and not let any external factors influence his internal calm. In fact, in chapter 2, verse 48, Krishna defines yoga as exactly that: equanimity.[1] As he exhorts Arjuna to live a life of balance, he explains that the devotees who live their lives undisturbed are the ones he loves most:

> He who neither disturbs
> the world nor is disturbed by it,
> who is free of all joy, fear, and envy—
> the man is the one I love best[2]

Krishna further defines his ideal devotee by describing them as "indifferent to praise and blame."[3] What Krishna is telling Arjuna is that to be equanimous, you have to have a certain level of control over two things: your emotions and how the world around you affects you.

Emotional fluctuations can be challenging to control. Consider that we do not all have the same amount of emotional intensity or resilience. Some people are more responsive to stimuli, and others seem more naturally removed from feelings of sadness, anxiety, or anger. (See chapter 26, on the doshas, for more discussion of our different natural constitutions.) If you feel like you struggle more than others with any of these harder emotions, offer yourself compassion—this part of you may be innate.

But even if it does seem like you naturally experience rage or despair more than your peers, part of your yoga practice is to grow more aware of this tendency and to begin to exercise control over how these emotions sway and disturb you. While it may not always feel like it in the immediate moment, how much energy or attention you give to each emotional fluctuation you experience is a choice.

In the West, there has been a movement toward welcoming more open emotionality in relation to embracing mental health. That's great! But sometimes, before you give into an emotional response, you might want to question the cause of the emotion. Any parent will tell you that although children's emotions are real and their feelings deeply matter, sometimes the cause of an outburst or outrage is a lack of sleep, too much sugar, or not enough quiet downtime. As adults, we are still vulnerable to responding to the world in bigger ways when we have not gotten our basic needs met. That doesn't make feelings of depression or anxiety any less real, but recognizing that your feelings might just be passing moments in response to unimportant stimuli can give you a little more perspective and space to choose whether to react from an emotional place or a place of equanimity.

Indeed, to not react from a place of emotion and to hold on to an inner sense of calm, undisturbed by events outside, is to move toward greater freedom. In *Man's Search for Meaning*, Viktor Frankl writes "Everything can be taken from a man but one thing: the last of the human freedoms—to choose one's attitude in any given set of circumstances, to choose one's own way."[4] When you arrive at a place where you can notice agitation or disruption to your inner peace and you can choose how to respond, you will feel more balanced both on and off the mat.

ACTIONS

Control your exposure to triggers. Does everyone have an estranged relative who posts vitriolic political messages and memes online? If you do, and it enrages you, please find the "block" button in your social media app as quickly as possible! While you cannot (and should not) hide from everything that you find emotionally challenging, you can make thoughtful decisions about your exposure to world news, talking heads, and any other media that relies on getting a rise out of you. Headlines are designed to distress you, piquing your interest so that you will read on. Don't take the bait: Scroll past it, block the account, or turn off the TV. If you find it hard to control your (understandable) sense of anger or despair at horrors in the world, remind yourself that you are not the only (or most important) witness, and limit your exposure to the triggers.

Take responsibility for your emotions. You might see this action as paradoxical to the first one, but it isn't; it's just a slightly different way to view things. Nothing (not your ranting Facebook uncle nor the disturbing YouTube video you just watched) is responsible for your emotions. You alone are in charge of those. Your partner, children, workplace, and friends exist in a world that connects to yours but does not control it. Resist the urge to blame outside forces for how you feel internally; remember Arjuna and be indifferent to praise and blame (and your children's frustrations and your partner's forgetfulness).

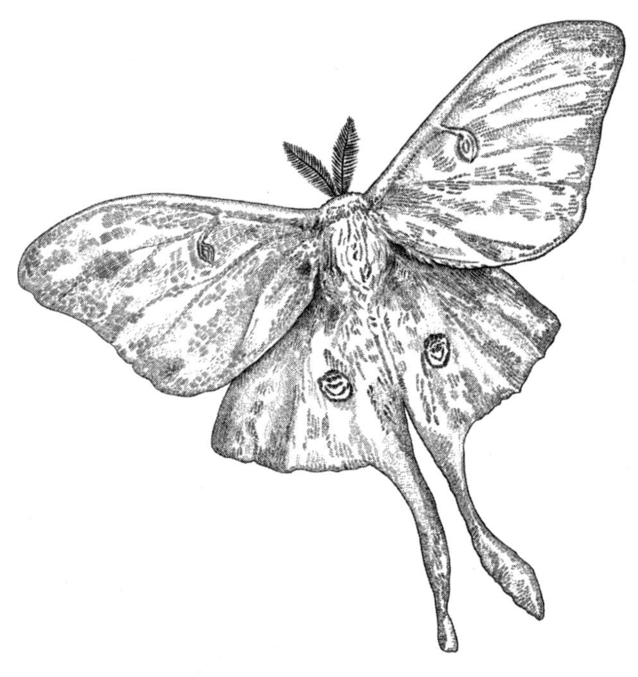

30
SELF AND MATTER

In much of yoga philosophy, there is a division between the Seen and the Seer, the Known and the Knower. In the introduction to this book, we talked about the varied history of yoga thought: In some moments it is dualist, and in others nondualist. When we consider the universe as *purusha* (the Seer, the Knower, pure consciousness) and *prakriti* (the Seen, the Known, all of material reality), we are describing a dualist philosophy.

Did we lose you yet? Here's another way to imagine it: Everything you can touch, feel, see, and understand is prakriti. Imagine a beautiful tree standing alone on a hillside. Prakriti is the tree and all parts of the tree: the fruit, the leaves, the branches, the bark, the trunk, the roots. But it's also everything around the tree: the grass, the soil, the sun, the water, the birds, insects—the very air around it!

Purusha, on the other hand, is the *why* in relation to the tree. Why does the tree exist in the first place? And why does it have fruit, leaves, and branches? Why is there grass and soil? *Why is there anything?*

Whether your answer to that is *God* or *I don't know*, you're right. That's sort of the point: Purusha is unknown, but omnipresent. Purusha is behind all of existence and completely intangible.

In other places in this book, we've described this division as Self (purusha) and matter (prakriti). When we describe purusha as "Self," it's commonplace to capitalize that word to distinguish it from the individual "self," as in oneself. But the Self of Purusha is that force (the God, the *why*) behind all of existence, including all of us, all the small-s selves.

ACTIONS

Trust that there is an answer. The idea that the universe is made up of everything we know and everything we don't implies that even where there is great mystery, there is still a plan in place. Max Ehrmann's 1927 poem "Desiderata" epitomizes this idea in the line "And whether or not it is clear to you, no doubt the universe is unfolding as it should." So does the Beatles' song lyric, "There will be an answer, let it be." Sitting with the ideas of purusha and prakriti means that you can allow the unknown to be a source of your continual faith in goodness, without having to determine exactly what those unknown things are.

Integrate the *what* and the *why*. Get curious, like a child who constantly asks, "Why? Why? Why?" When you see or hear something interesting in the natural world—a moth you've never seen before, a cloud formation that's new to you, a whispering wall inside a canyon or a dome—investigate it more fully. What is there to see? What is there to feel, if it's a tangible thing? To hear, to smell, even to taste? This is honing your attunement to prakriti.

Then, once you've collected as much data as you can about the *what*, investigate the *why*. There may not be an immediate answer, or any answer, but there could be—a quick internet search can explain why luna moths don't have functional mouths, or what weather pattern caused that saucer-shaped cloud, or how dome architecture amplifies sound. The more you tune in to the *why*, the more you align with the universe.

31

MASCULINE AND FEMININE

As we've seen, there's a tension throughout yoga philosophy between binary or dualist thinking, where two categories exist independently of each other (like *purusha* and *prakriti*), and nonbinary, nondualist thinking, where everything is part of the one. Yoga philosophy frequently guides us to find the delicate balance between two competing energies, attitudes, or actions. For example, in this book we've already explored:

- *asteya* and *aparigraha* (not stealing and not hoarding)

- *tapas* and *Ishvara pranidhana* (dedication and surrender)

- *abhyasa* and *vairagya* (action and dispassion)

- *prana vayu* and *apana vayu* (rising and falling energy)

- *samana vayu* and *vyana vayu* (concentrating and expanding energy)

- *rajasic* and *tamasic* gunas (action and inertia)

If this still feels esoteric, let's consider a concept we're all familiar with, as it's been applied to us since before birth: masculine and feminine energies. Different cultures, at different times, have reconciled these energies as both binary and nonbinary.

One approach yoga philosophy has used to describe this balance comes from Hindu mythology, in which Shiva and Shakti are avatars of these two energies. Shiva is the masculine; his wife, Shakti, is the feminine. They are sometimes depicted as one figure, Ardhanarishvara: a half-male, half-female being that unites the qualities of both. (While Shiva and Shakti are the most commonly used names for these deities, in tantric texts like the *Bhairava Tantra* they show up as Bhairava (masculine) and Devi (feminine).) The dynamic of Shiva and Shakti might suggest dualism, reminiscent of purusha and prakriti, but the difference is that while purusha and prakriti are seen as separate, coexisting things, Shiva and Shakti are two halves that form a singular whole.

If we think of the gendered experience as a complete sphere, where things are roughly half male and half female, there is still not a clear determination in where the dividing line is. This is how we see gender play out in energetic forms. Whether you are born into a body assigned as a woman or a man (and whether you ultimately feel that your gender conforms with that body), you are made of and act from a place of both masculine and feminine energies. You are composed of both Shiva and Shakti.

Hindu stories serve as beautiful examples of yoga; after all, Hinduism developed alongside yoga, in the same region of the world. That's why we often see Hindu iconography used to represent yogic themes. In story after story, Shiva and Shakti teach us about union and separation, as well as creation and destruction, but at the heart of their stories is their need for one another in order to form a more complete whole.

Masculine and feminine energy abides in all of us. You need both of these energies—though perhaps in different proportions than others—to be your whole self.

ACTIONS

Get in touch with your masculine or feminine side. What do you think of as inherently masculine traits? Feminine traits? Your age, culture, and upbringing probably determine your answer to that. And that's just fine: We don't all have to agree on a set of stereotypes for men and women. What's important for this exercise is that *you* determine what is "masculine" and what is "feminine" in yourself. How do you channel these energies? Maybe you already define yourself as a "sensitive man," but your interpretation of "sensitivity" could be a masculine trait or a feminine one. Or maybe you see yourself as a "powerful woman," but your interpretation of "powerful" could have feminine or masculine energy. Maybe your expressions of gendered experience look quite different from those examples. But take a moment to investigate how the spectrum of gender is expressed in your actions, choices, and appearance. Consider whether you want to express any gendered traits more than you already are in your daily life.

Get more creative. All of us need more creative outlets, especially in purpose-driven, Western societies where achievement, typically understood as a masculine energy, rules the culture. Creativity and creation, in contrast, are usually seen as the domain of femininity. One way you can bring more Shakti energy into your life is to create without a guiding reason or greater purpose. Allow your creative energy to bring you to passionate art-making, ecstatic dancing, and loud bathroom singing—without a need for any of it to be tied to achievement, perfection, or even completion. This type of creativity should be guided by your intuition and impulses.

32

EFFORT AND EASE

Balancing *sthira* (effort) and *sukha* (ease) is at the heart of a yoga asana practice. But sthira and sukha also guide how we walk through our daily life. We want to be friendly and warm, but also powerful. We want to be compassionate, but also strong. We want to be flexible, but also principled.

Finding this balance is a constant quest. Just when you think you've achieved the perfect equilibrium, life throws you a curve ball and you get out of whack. But achieving some ideal balanced state is an impossibility. It's all in the work of getting closer to it, yet never fully achieving it.

A major benefit of practicing yoga on and off the mat is honing your discernment to recognize when effort is appropriate and when ease is called for, when it's time to bear down and when it's time to ease off, when it's time to push and when it's time to pull. In the words of the gambler in that old Kenny Rogers song, "You've got to know when to hold 'em, know when to fold 'em."

But this is not something you inherently know in all situations and circumstances. That's why you learn from practice. We know this to be true in our asana practice. If you've practiced physical yoga long enough, you've almost inevitably had an experience where you pushed a challenging pose a little too far and found yourself injured. But you've also undoubtedly had the experience of attaining a pose, through persistence and practice, that had at first seemed impossible. (That first wall-free handstand probably felt pretty amazing.)

You have to apply this same practice to your yoga off the mat, remembering that you won't always get it right on the first try. If you find yourself at an impasse, in a situation that will not budge despite your repeated attempts at action, it may be time for *inaction*, for ease, for surrender. And, on the other hand, when you find that you are not growing, not evolving, or not developing more fully toward your true, divine Self, it's time for action.

ACTIONS

Meditate. There is no better place to explore the application of effort and ease than in meditation. Maybe you already have a meditation practice in place, or maybe this is something you'd like to begin. Effort and ease are the twin energies of meditation. You must put in enough effort that you stay awake, alert, and connected to an anchor for your wandering attention (like your breath, a mantra, or a candle flame). But you also must stay relaxed, bringing enough ease and softness to the practice to allow it to unfold without expectation. The next time you come to sit in meditation, allow yourself to notice the precise balance of effort and ease required for the practice. Every successful session is setting up the next one.

Ask a trusted loved one. Aside from yourself, there is probably a person in your life—a trusted partner or best friend—who is familiar with where you tend to be too lax and where you metaphorically bang your head against a wall with unnecessary force. Start a conversation with this person about your desire for creating balance between effort and ease in your life. Ask them: *Where do I try too hard? Where should I be putting in more time or energy?* You might be surprised to find that they have an easy answer you wouldn't have thought of.

33

DISCIPLINE IS FREEDOM

Having the discipline to practice yoga—especially practicing on your own, when you are accountable only to yourself and your Self—can feel like an enormous effort. But when we perceive disciplined living as an opportunity for freedom, we find ease.

When you were a teenager, you likely bristled against the constraints your parents, teachers, and society put on you. You couldn't *wait* to be free of the rigid schedule, the chores and apparent busywork, the demand for conformity. But now that you're older, you might dream of a routine where other people take on the duty of decision-making, and of a life where you know just what is expected of you and what the metrics of success look like! Like a retired soldier who still makes the bed to military standards, you might as an adult choose to lean into disciplined habits that turn out to be a source of freedom.

Freedom? How? Because these disciplined habits (tapas) actually free you from the petty decision-making that can eat up much of your energy and attention every day. When you develop discipline, you don't have to wonder whether or where or how or when to meditate; instead, you know that you *will* meditate daily; it happens on your cushion facing the back yard; it involves repeating your mantra for twenty minutes; and it happens after you rise and before you get the coffee brewing. Freed from the effort of working through a decision tree every day just to get onto your meditation cushion, your mind is better able to settle into the here and now and the act of sitting. Your routine frees you from indecision or paralysis.

Even better, when you hone your presence, focus, and awareness in this daily meditation, it becomes easier to continue the disciplined practice of self-study across every moment of your day, using the techniques you've read here (and any others that make sense to you). So if you're coming to the end of this book excited to make a daily habit of yoga practice off the mat, discipline is your natural ally. We offer some scaffolding to help you build that discipline in part VI.

ACTIONS

Make a small commitment—and keep it. Is there some aspect of yoga that eludes you? For instance, maybe you find meditation a challenge. Make a commitment to include this aspect of yoga in your life in a small way. Decide that for this week only, you'll meditate for five minutes every night before bed. Then set a "meditation reminder" notification on your phone; when the alarm goes off, just do it, without thinking about it twice. Notice the freedom this act of discipline creates.

One step at a time. Even if you're really excited to try all of the actions in this book, you'll ultimately develop a deeper, more sustainable practice if you start small. Think about bite-sized chunks, not bingeable feasts. Maybe you start with just *one* of the actions we suggested in chapter 1, not all of them. Or better yet, start with the one action that feels closest to something you already naturally do. Then keep building from there. Maybe you'll add one a day, or one a week. There's no real goal here—beyond the enormous goal of knowing yourself as divine and finding union, balance, and connection through yoga. But this can happen with one little action step done regularly over time. That might even get you there faster than trying to complete every single action in this book, getting a fifth of the way in, and quitting. We like to imagine our readers using this book as a guide to intention-setting; you can come back to it whenever you are feeling like you're straying from your spiritual path and find suggestions that help you back onto it.

34

SAMENESS

If you've got an ear for language, you may have noticed the word *sama*, meaning "same" or "evenness," turns up a lot in your yoga class. For example, one description of mountain pose is *samastithi*, standing steady. When we unite via yoga, either as a community practicing together in a class or as a personal practice that yokes together consciousness and matter, soul and body, we experience a great sameness—*samyama*. The playing field becomes more level, flatter. We become equal. We lose the illusion that we are separate from other beings, and we see the divine spark in all of us.

You may have felt this in collective gatherings, like concerts, plays, or sporting events, where everyone is sharing the same experience. Or, if you run, perhaps you've felt it in the context of a race, where you were striving to reach the finish line in an apparent competition with others, but the effort unleashed a sense of connection and oneness. At the other end of human experience, maybe you've felt that connection while sitting at someone's deathbed, watching hospice workers treat everyone, patient and family, with loving-kindness. Maybe you have found this sense of union in your own yoga practice, or breath work, or meditation. For many readers of this book, we wager you sense this sameness at the end of a yoga class.

Two phrases you might have heard in yoga class point to this. One is the once-typical ending of yoga class: *Namaste.* The literal translation of the greeting is "not-me to you." It's a gesture of deferential respect and humility. As you may have experienced in a Western yoga class, some teachers will say a whole poem about *namaste* as a concept, along the lines of, "The light in me sees and honors the light in you, and when we are in that place, we are one." This interpretation goes afield of the traditional translation of *namaste* and of its current usage in South Asia, where it is more of a "hello" than a "goodbye." (With increased sensitivity about cultural appropriation, some teachers, including us, have dropped the term in class.) However, the intention of the poetic interpretation is lovely and points directly to the union that yoga promises: a sense of shared experience, sameness, and collective connection.

Another common class ending is this mantra, often chanted at closing or expressed in English as a prayer: *Lokah samastha sukhino bhavantu.* The meaning is "May all beings (*samastha*) in the place (*lokah*) have a feeling (*bhav*) of ease and freedom (*sukhino*)." Similar to the explosion of *namaste* into a full poem, in the West this message usually has some addenda tacked on: "And may my thoughts, words, and deeds contribute to the happiness and freedom of all beings." Again, this is a beautiful description of our shared experience of both humanity and divinity, and it points to our interconnection and interdependence. What better message to leave your mat with than the injunction to act in a way that contributes to liberation for all?

ACTIONS

See the light in everyone. Take the poetic interpretation of *namaste* off your mat and into the world. Greet people as the embodiment of the divine that they are. Recognize that everyone you encounter over the course of the day shares a desire for happiness and freedom, just as you do. Operate from this assumption and greet everyone with love, so that the light in you sees and honors the light in them. See if this act of reflecting others' light back at them doesn't make your own day brighter!

Live the prayer. Use the concept of sameness as a filter: Before you think, speak, and act, remember our shared connection and the similarity between all beings. Can you apply the Golden Rule, and treat your equal as yourself? Can you treat others exactly as you would like to be treated? Ultimately, your actions toward anyone are your actions toward *everyone*, including yourself. How can you live your life so that your existence is a step toward happiness and freedom for all beings?

35

THE LESSON OF LETTING

The main lesson of the Bhagavad Gita might be summarized, "Do your duty with no attachment to results." The question then becomes, "What is your duty?" For Arjuna in the Bhagavad Gita, it was to be a brave warrior. In our modern, complicated lives, we often owe allegiance or have responsibilities to more than one person. You may be a partner or spouse and also a parent (to humans or four-legged kids). You might additionally be a friend, a sibling, a child, or a colleague. In all of these roles, there is duty. And in all of these roles, it's highly tempting to attach that duty to some specific, expected outcome.

Consider the role of a parent and the work inherent in that role. A parent is responsible for being kind and loving, setting appropriate boundaries, and offering comfort and support. As parents ourselves, we know that the work of parenting is often a thankless task—especially the first few hands-on, low-sleep years. But as parents, we don't love our children as part of a specific plan that leads to a certain outcome. We don't nurture our children with an end goal in mind. Instead, we adore and celebrate our children because that's our duty as parents. Doing that duty feels good, and it's how it's supposed to be—regardless of who our children become or how they turn out. That part is out of our hands.

This understanding is not an easy one to arrive at. Often, we do our duty in a role with an end result in mind, either consciously or unconsciously. For instance, you might expect reciprocation when you do something kind for your partner. You might expect praise when you go above or beyond in your workplace. The key word in this is *expect*. To do your duty with no attachment to results is to deeply comprehend the truth at hand: What is in your control is only ever your own actions. Anyone else's actions are *not* in your control. When you know that to be true, you move in the world concerned only with your own duty. You allow. You let.

ACTIONS

Temper your expectations. Have you ever tried something for the first time with the expectation that it may not be your cup of tea? In these situations, you might be joyfully surprised by the fun you have. When you have low (or better, no) expectations, you're not seeking out a specific result. You can apply this when you try a new restaurant, take a trip to a place you've never been, or sit down to watch a recommended movie. What expectations do you have? How do these expectations set you up to expect certain results? Can you try this restaurant, go on vacation, or watch the movie without projecting an expectation onto the experience?

Question your disappointments. Similarly, take some time to catalog your biggest disappointments. You might journal about this, writing about a job you wish you'd taken or a relationship you wish you'd walked away from sooner. Notice that within many of these disappointments is a sense of wanting *someone else* to have acted differently. Look again at these disappointments. With fresh perspective, can you see your disappointments as attachment to expected results?

PART VI

LIVING YOUR YOGA

Ideas aren't worth much unless they are put into action. That's why each of the chapters in parts I through V offers you a few actions or steps to take so that you can *live* your yoga. It's only through conscious implementation of these concepts that you'll come to understand them. No amount of book knowledge will replace lived experience or the resonance that comes from an idea moved into action with intention. Let's explore what you can do to enact what you've learned. In this part, we'll discuss how you can continue to process yoga philosophy to feel better connected, balanced, and more free, as well as how you can keep learning more about yoga off the mat.

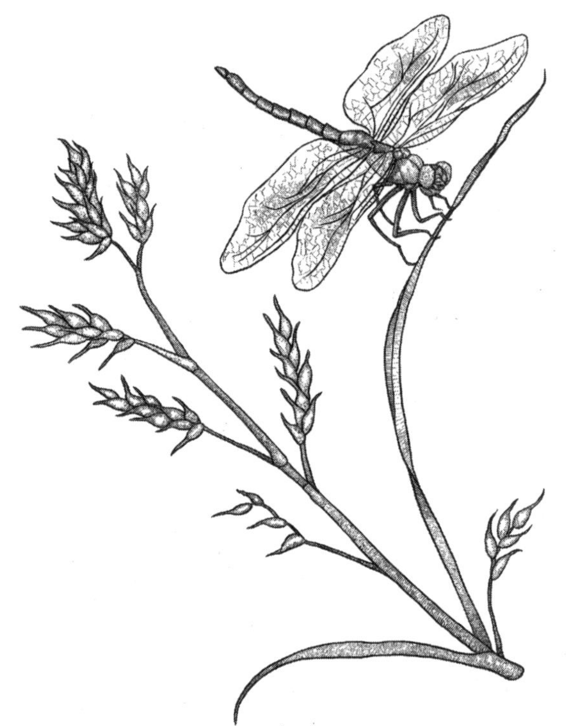

36

SAMPLE SCHEDULES

We don't want to micromanage your yoga practice, either on the mat or off it. We aren't here to insist that your knee stays directly over your ankle in a lunge, your heels reach the ground in downward-facing dog, and your tailbone angle is *just so* in chair pose. You do you. Similarly, we aren't here to demand that you develop a daily habit of reading yogic texts, sound-cleansing your chakras, and doing selfless service. If you feel inspired by your deepening practice and understanding of yoga concepts to do this, fantastic! There may be plenty of concepts in this book that you can't wait to see come alive in your life. But that impetus must come from inside you, not from any teacher—and certainly not from any sample schedule in a book.

In keeping with this nondogmatic approach, there also may be some ideas that don't resonate with you (now or ever), which you can leave behind. The purpose of this book is to offer you many philosophical ideas to explore so that you can find the ones that feel most salient to your life now.

However, we know it can be helpful to have some scaffolding on which to hang your ongoing practice of yoga, especially as you explore some of the ideas you've read about in this book. So in this chapter, we give you some tangible ways to take your yoga off the mat and into your day, week, month, and year, whether you spend one minute per day on it or an hour. Please take everything here as a simple suggestion. Run with what works for you and leave the rest behind with no guilt.

Things You Can Do In. . .

ONE MINUTE

- Take three slow, intentional breaths to be in the now.

- Practice a one-minute *pratyahara* meditation: Rub your hands together to warm them, then place them in turn over your eyes, your ears, and your nose and mouth (lightly), followed by your heart and your belly, or rest them on your lap. As you do, drop in and away from the information you'd been processing through your senses of sight, hearing, smell, taste, and touch. Listen for the inner voice.

- Posit at least one alternative hypothesis for a vexing situation.

- Greet a stranger with love. Don't go overboard; just step outside your own agenda and busy schedule, take a deep breath, make eye contact, and say a meaningful hello.

- Before taking an action of kindness—sending a thank-you email, letting someone cut the line at the grocery, donating to charity—take a moment to consciously release your attachment to the results of your action. Let the action exist solely as an expression of love, not as a signal of your virtue or need for recognition.

- Find some small way to impose order (*saucha*) on your physical surroundings: Move a stack of junk mail into recycling, or clear up your virtual desktop.

- Practice *santosha* by finding something you feel especially grateful about in your life, as it is at this very moment.

- In the spirit of bringing more *sattva* into your life, reminisce about a moment of joy and light from the past few weeks.

- If you notice your mind wandering or jumping from thought to thought, label the sort of thoughts you're having. Are they memories? Are you working through a complex thought? Are you spending time imagining things?

FIVE MINUTES

- Have a spontaneous dance party! Put on your favorite tune and move your body. Try not to execute any "official" dance moves or yoga poses. Be a vessel for the playful expression of the universe. Channel Shakti and lila.

- Chant on your own. Take a few minutes to vocalize whatever sound wants to come through you. This can be as simple as expressing an enormous sigh (*ahhhhhh*) or an *om,* or it can be as complex as chanting a mantra (like *lokah samastha sukhino bhavantu* or your own personal favorite Sanskrit mantra). It can also be powerful to sing a song aloud (but only to and for yourself) that has deep meaning to you.

- Set a timer for five minutes and look through one drawer of clothing, or one section of your closet, or the furniture in one room of your house. What could you be hoarding (unintentionally, perhaps) that could be of use to others? Follow *aparigraha* and set it aside to donate.

- Leave five minutes earlier than you typically do for your next meeting, so as not to steal others' time.

- Set a timer for five minutes and then step away from any devices. Do whatever you want in this time: stretch, lie in the sun, let your mind wander. Give yourself a moment to be free from doing.

- Scroll, but scroll mindfully. Look for things that make you laugh, smile, and feel connected to humanity. Comment with kind enthusiasm.

- Walk outside. Look at the trees, the grass, a spider's web. Allow time in the natural world to revitalize you and remind you of the magic inherent in existence.

- Read a poem. We love the bite-size beauty that small amounts of gorgeous writing can offer. You may find something particularly resonant in the work of poets we love, and who often appear as suggestions for yoga inspiration: Wendell Berry, Mary Oliver, Rumi, Hafez, Thich Nhat Hanh, Derek Walcott, Jane Hirschfield, or Alice Walker.

THIRTY MINUTES

- Thirty minutes gives you time for meditation and journaling. Choose a focus of your meditation—a mantra, your breath, a physical object—and spend twenty minutes sitting, followed by ten minutes writing.

- Commit to an act of service. Pick up roadside trash. Help an elder load their groceries into the trunk of their car, and take the time to connect with them and ask about their day. Drop off some treats at the fire department. No matter what you do, be sure you are acting without attachment to the results—without needing to be seen doing good works.

- Do something that's uncomfortable for you, like going for a jog or taking a cold shower. Notice this challenging act for what it is: discomfort, but not suffering.

- Lie on the floor and feel your way through the koshas: Start with your physical body and move through your breath body, your thinking body, your intuitive body, and your bliss body.

- Choose a chakra to immerse yourself in. Bring the color of that chakra into this immersion, perhaps through the clothing you wear or through a coloring exercise. Ask yourself questions about this chakra to see what you uncover, and practice chanting the mantra sound associated with it.

- Learn about your dosha. If you haven't taken a quiz to determine your dosha, do that first. Then read about your dosha type, noting whether you feel your dosha is in or out of balance.

- Move your body in a free-flowing way, whether that's dancing or walking or yoga. As you move, try things out: Raise your arms or do a little hop. Notice not just the physical movements but also how prana courses through your body and limbs.

SIXTY MINUTES

- Read scripture or other inspiring writing carefully for twenty minutes. Then set it down and spend twenty minutes in seated contemplation or meditation—or, alternatively, move your body as a way to process what you've read. Spend the next twenty minutes journaling about the experience, without needing to arrive at any particular conclusion.

- Do some calendar cleanout. Look at your schedule with an eye to how you've been spending your time and how you would *like* to be spending your time. If you see events or commitments that are preventing you from living a balanced life—from finding a sattvic harmony between work and leisure, duty and play—take some steps to restore the balance. Resign from a committee. Say no to requests that don't align with your higher purpose.

Then fill the white space in your calendar with placeholders to work through some of the other suggestions in this chapter or to do whatever most brings you a sense of joy, connection, and freedom.

- Be a klesha hunter: In conjunction with a skilled therapist or a friend who knows you well, take an hour to explore where the kleshas—wrong-seeing, ego, craving, aversion, and fear—are holding you back. Jointly imagine a life for yourself that is free from some of the suffering these patterns have been causing. Brainstorm how you might release yourself from these habits and forge new ones that will move you toward freedom.

- Identify a vasana or samskara—something that has you stuck. A good starting point is a tough memory. Imagine moments from a difficult time in your life. Or you could literally take out or pull up photos from that time. Notice how you look and who else is in the pictures with you. Notice, too, that the you in these past images is both you and not you. Consider how this tough memory still guides your actions (or inactions). Is it time for a change?

Actions You Might Take . . .

DAILY

- Build a short but regular period of meditation into your day. Even five minutes done with regularity can contribute immensely to your personal sense of well-being. Mark it on your calendar and set yourself a reminder, then lean into the ease of this discipline.

- Check in with yourself to clearly see the state of your being. How balanced do you feel your energies are today? If something feels out of whack, what would it take to come back toward harmony?

- Get inspiration from any yogic text; we have a list for you at the end of the book. Set it next to your bedside and read rather than scroll at the end or beginning of your day.

- Establish a clear morning routine that aligns with your energetic intent. Need more rajas? Get up earlier. Craving the groundedness of tamas? Turn off your alarm. Determine what routine in the morning allows you to ultimately feel most sattvic as the day unfolds.

- Develop a nightly metta practice. As you lie in bed, send loving-kindness to friends, loved ones, and the world outside of yourself. Much like a gratitude list, a daily metta practice will increase your sense of joy and belonging.

- Get clear about your duty. If your goal is to emulate Arjuna and do your duty with no attachment to results, you have to fully understand what your duty is, specific to the different relationships and contexts in your life. What's your duty on a Monday morning, heading into your office? What's your duty in relation to your child's school or your neighborhood? Define your duty daily, so you're clear on the scope of your purpose in relation to the day.

WEEKLY

- Choose one model from part IV to explore each week: the koshas, bandhas, chakras, doshas, vayus, or gunas. You might reread the corresponding chapter and practice the suggested actions. Devise your own practice that explores one or all of the elements of this model, as you understand it. As you work with this concept, how does it inform your asana practice, and vice versa?

  - Stay attuned to this energy as you move through your week. Where is it manifest in your experience? In your actions? In the actions of others?

- You could even slow it down further than that and investigate each kosha or chakra over the course of a week. How would it feel to focus on anahata chakra for an entire week? What would that look like?

- There are fifty-two weeks in a year. Are there fifty-two angles or elements of yoga that you want to grow deeper in? Could you map out an investigation of one a week? Keep in mind that you don't have to adhere to this exact goal over the course of just one year, since these demarcations of time are arbitrary!

- Be very clear on what constitutes the start of your week, and set aside some sacred time to prepare for the week ahead. We don't mean meal-prepping or writing out your to-do list. We mean considering your spiritual needs for the week ahead. What does that look like? Maybe it looks like no action, just awareness. Or maybe it looks like scheduling out your meditation or yoga time in advance.

- Set up a Sattvic Social. Once a week, spend time with a friend, acquaintance, or mentor who inspires you to be your best self—have lunch or tea, or go for a walk.

MONTHLY

- Attend a yoga workshop, kirtan, or ecstatic dance.

- Attend a spiritual gathering: a religious service, a celebration of life, a baptism, or the regular services of another faith. Show up with an open mind and heart and the intention to find common ground. (Sage was given this assignment in a religion class in college, and it made an impression on her that lingers to this day.)

  - There's no need to write a lengthy paper about your experience, but if you'd like to journal about it, even better.

  - More bonus points for accompanying a friend to a meeting or service of their own faith or spiritual practice, be it shabbat or a 12-step meeting.

- Set a monthly *atha* check-in. Once a month, set aside time for self-reflection that is specific to your yogic or spiritual path. Are you here now? What's pulling you off your path? How are you, really?

- Explore your shadow. Once a month, ask hard questions about the kleshas and what hidden obstacles are guiding you. Maybe create a "shadow evening" once a month, spending time alone with your journal, seeing things as they truly are—and considering what you'd like to change.

- Commit to a yogic text. That could be an ancient text or a modern revision of yogic ideas. Buy the book, read the book, and move through it in a month. That's twelve books a year to open your eyes and help you cultivate freedom. We have suggestions in References and Further Study on page 185.

- Once a month, watch something sattvic. Rather than your usual Netflix binge or true-crime favorite, watch a nature documentary, or a movie about success against the odds, or any show that helps you remember and believe in the good in the world. We have ideas for this in References and Further Study on page 185.

ANNUALLY

- Schedule a retreat. Depending on your budget and time, this can be a formal visit to a retreat center, a destination experience, or a DIY staycation. The point is not the setting, but rather the intention to withdraw and spend time in self-study and contemplation. Create a scenario in which you can unplug in a way that feels spacious, not unmooring. This might mean a few phone-free hours a day or a complete ten-day silent retreat. Go just beyond the edges of your comfort zone, so you're stretching but not setting yourself up for failure.

- Make sure your holiday rituals align with your yogic ideals. Maybe it's time to give up the all-night new year's event in exchange for a yoga mala at your local studio. Your birthday is another annual holiday that can become an opportunity for deepening your practice off the mat. Rather than spending your birthday fully with others, maybe use it as a silent day, walk in nature, or spend time without electronics.

- Celebrate all the New Year holidays: Chinese New Year, Rosh Hashanah, Nav Varsh, and the Gregorian calendar new year of January 1. Use holidays with the spirit of new beginning to have a regular check-in with yourself throughout your year. This allows you to deepen your mindfulness and self-awareness but also to learn more about cultural celebrations that may not be your own. (And yes, we know this is technically not an "annual" practice!)

- Celebrate other holidays that feel spiritually relevant, even if they are culturally foreign. In Alexandra's house, they celebrate Dia de los Muertos. While this holiday is celebrated widely in Mexico and other parts of Latin America, it may not be familiar to you. Dia de los Muertos gives celebrants a chance to remember their dead loved ones. Altars are made, favorite foods are prepared, and memories are shared. Get curious about how other cultures commemorate the vicissitudes of life—you might find a new perspective and a new way into the divine.

37

PHILOSOPHICAL PROMPTS

Here are some suggestions for your contemplation, based on some of the concepts in this book. You might like to journal about these, or to choose one to sit with—or walk, or run, or practice asanas with—for a session, a day, or a week at a time. These questions may serve as intentions for your yoga practice on or off the mat.

The Yamas and the Niyamas

Ahimsa: In what ways could you reduce your harm footprint in life? How could this happen physically? Emotionally? Environmentally?

Satya: Where are you most honest, both with yourself and others? Where do you have a tendency to hold back from honesty, and why? Do you stray from the path of honesty out of an urge to protect yourself? To protect others?

Asteya: What do you covet that isn't yours? Where do you take more than you need?

Brahmacharya: What is the right energy for right now? For a major task ahead? How can you ensure you find the best balance between taking only what you need and sharing everything you can?

Aparigraha: What resources do you have that could benefit others—material resources, financial resources, or your time? How can you share them more freely?

Saucha: Where do you tend toward disorder in your life? How can you clean up your act—physically, emotionally, or otherwise?

Santosha: What would it take to be happy right here, right now, with nothing changing externally? What shifts can you take to practice equanimity and contentment? What field of focus do you need for this—is it a macroscope, zooming way out to see that your existence is a drop in the divine ocean? Is it a microscope, narrowing your attention into a single breath, or even a single inhale or exhale?

Tapas: Where in your life does discipline come easily to you? Where do you find it difficult to toe the line? What would change if you applied more effort and enthusiasm in the tough spots?

Svadhyaya: What kind of introspection comes easily to you? For example, are you responding to these prompts by journaling, or by thinking about them during your daily walk? Where do you find it difficult to take an honest look at yourself? Where does your yoga practice fit into this mix?

Ishvara Pranidhana: What if you just let go? What does it look like to have the serenity to accept the things you cannot change?

The Five Kleshas

Consider a time when you had the wrong view of things. Is there anything in your life now that is being understood incorrectly because of avidya?

Knowing that your ego drives most of your interactions, can you identify a place in your life where you would like asmita to take the backseat?

Raga and dvesha are ultimately about expectations and desires. This can lead to unnecessary suffering. The irony is that a lot of the suffering comes from small things that don't ultimately matter that much. Can you think of places in your life you could do a better job of not sweating the small stuff to reduce your suffering?

Does a fear of the unknown drive any of your habits? Do you feel like you have enough time to do everything you want to do and see everything you want to see?

Balancing Your Energies

What do you most desire? Where in your body do you feel this craving? How long does it last when it sets in?

What do you most detest? Where in your body do you feel this aversion? How long does it last when it sets in?

When do you feel sluggish, slow, or filled with inertia? Is it keyed to the calendar, weather, work, your diet, or something else?

When do you feel steady, grounded, deliberate, and resolved? What circumstances contribute to this?

When do you feel uptight, anxious, scattered, and ungrounded? What circumstances contribute to this?

When do you feel creative, free, and full of lightness? What circumstances contribute to this?

When do you feel irritated, angry, and inflamed? What circumstances contribute to this?

When do you feel powerful, ready to get things done, and ready to move and shake? What circumstances contribute to this?

When, where, and with whom do you feel impelled to action? When is effort the best path? What circumstances contribute to this, and what enhances this feeling?

When, where, and with whom do you feel ready to let go? When do you feel at ease? What circumstances contribute to this, and what enhances this feeling?

Do you feel like your actions and attitude are gendered in a specific way? What shifts could you make to bring in more Shakti or Shiva energy and create greater harmony?

Deep Conditioning

Write about a habit of yours. It may be wise to start small, with something you might feel like changing but that isn't causing major problems in your life—for example, a habit of eating a handful of Skittles after every lunch at home. (Yes, we're speaking from personal experience here; lime is the best flavor.) Can you trace the origins of this habit back to your earliest memory of it? What made this habit useful then? What keeps it useful now? What would your experience be if you chose a new habit?

Write about a habit of yours that both yields positive results and feels easy for you to do—for example, making the bed every morning. Think about what other habits you might be able to stack onto this one: Maybe you make the bed, then sit on its edge and take five mindful breaths. Create a plan to try this for a week. If you like the results, try layering another habit into the stack.

Chart out the parts of you that are self and the parts of you that are Self. It might be helpful to draw a Venn diagram showing where they overlap, since certainly some parts are both. Can you ascribe less relevance to the small-s self parts?

Create a ritual that makes you feel divine. Write it out: Does it need to happen at a specific time of day? Do you need certain foods or activities? Do you conduct this ritual alone or with others? Does the ritual draw from other traditions? Explain the specifics of the ritual, its significance to you, and the mystical quality that drives it.

Elements of Your Being

Sit quietly and feel the state of being in your body now. Can you identify any of the concepts we explored in part IV and part V at play? Where in your body, mind, or spirit do you feel them? What is that experience like? Does it have a sensation, color, sound, word, or thought associated with it?

Draw images that capture your experience of and associations with the chakras. As you draw, tune in to each of the chakras, bottom to top. In the spirit of creating art with no goal, resist judgment or concern regarding what you create: Simply create, and let the act of creating help you learn about yourself.

Create a yoga-asana sequence for each of the vayus. What movements feel like they encourage apana vayu? Prana vayu? Udana, samana, and vyana vayu? This practice reminds you to tune into your subtle body, to notice how physical movement feels energetically.

Write out a metta list, where you list all the people and beings in your life that you love and value, and explain why you love and value them. Focus on the good you already have in your life, and see it grow.

Create an image of freedom, using some artistic medium—it could be a poem, drawing, or abstract painting. What does liberation look like to you? How can you capture that feeling in a piece of art?

Do less. Just sit, without an agenda—even a meditative one. It's enough to witness yourself existing and recognize the magic and mysticism inherent in that.

ACKNOWLEDGMENTS

Thanks to you, the reader, for your presence and attention here. The more people who are interested in yoga's gifts of self-improvement, connection, and freedom, the better off we all are.

Thanks to our agent, Linda Konner. Thanks to Shayna Keyles, Jasmine Respess, and Janelle Ludowise at North Atlantic Books; to copyeditor Erin Wiegand, whose careful attention vastly improved our work; to proofreader Chuck Hutchinson; to cover designer Jasmine Hromjak; and to the typesetter Maureen Forys.

Special thanks to Lasha Mutual for contributing her art once again—this is our third book graced by her illustrations. Lasha is able to evoke deep philosophical lessons nonverbally but profoundly, just with the stroke of a digital pen.

Thanks to our students in North Carolina and around the world for being earnest seekers who want to unite with the divine within.

Thanks most of all to our families and to our special partnership, which makes completing projects like this always feel like less than half the work—and more than double the fun.

GLOSSARY

abhinivesha Fear of the unknown; the fifth klesha, often translated as fear of death or clinging to life.

ahimsa Nonviolence; the first yama, directing practitioners to avoid violence and harm to others and to themselves.

ajna The third-eye chakra (indigo), located between the eyebrows; governs intuition and insight.

anahata The heart chakra (green), located at the heart space; governs relationships, forgiveness, trust, empathy, and generosity.

anandamaya kosha The bliss body; the innermost of the five koshas, representing one's true radiant nature.

annamaya kosha The physical sheath; the outermost of the five koshas, the densest and most superficial layer.

aparigraha Nonhoarding; the fifth yama, instructing practitioners not to amass more than they need.

asana Seat or physical posture, which should be both steady and comfortable; the third limb of yoga.

asmita Ego; the second klesha, caused by attachment to the small self and the illusion of separateness.

asteya Nonstealing; the third yama, reminding practitioners not to take what is not theirs, including time and energy.

atha "And now"; the opening word of the Yoga Sutras, a rhetorical call to presence in the immediate moment.

avidya Wrong-seeing or misperception; the first and root klesha, from which other obstacles arise.

bandhas Energetic locks in the body that help control the flow of prana.

Bhagavad Gita An important yogic text presenting a conversation between Krishna and Arjuna on the battlefield.

brahmacharya Temperance; the fourth yama, asking practitioners to use their personal energy responsibly.

chakras Energetic centers in the subtle body where the ida and pingala nadis cross; typically understood as seven centers from the base of the spine to the crown of the head.

chitta The mind or consciousness.

dharana Single-pointed concentration; the sixth limb of yoga, focusing attention on one thing.

dhyana Meditative awareness or presence in the moment; the seventh limb of yoga.

doshas The three constitutional types in Ayurveda, which describe inherent qualities and tendencies.

drishti Setting your gaze on a nonmoving object; a tool to help sustain attention during meditation or asana practice.

dvesha Aversion; one of the twin kleshas (with raga), the desire for something present to go away.

gunas The three qualities of nature—sattva (balance), rajas (excitation), and tamas (lethargy).

ida The main left energetic channel (nadi) in the subtle body, spiraling around the central sushumna nadi.

Ishvara pranidhana Surrender to the divine; the fifth niyama, asking practitioners to recognize something bigger than themselves.

kaivalya Liberation or absolute freedom.

kleshas The five obstacles to full realization—avidya, asmita, raga, dvesha, and abhinivesha.

koshas The five sheaths or layers of being, from the gross physical body to the subtle bliss body.

kundalini Higher spiritual consciousness that rises from its origin at the base of the spine to the crown of the head.

manipura The solar-plexus chakra (yellow), located at the navel; governs self-esteem and personal power.

manomaya kosha The thinking and feeling sheath; the layer of thoughts, moods, wants, and needs.

mantra A repeated phrase or sound used to sustain attention during meditation.

maya The illusion of separateness from divinity, which causes attachment to the material world.

moksha Liberation or freedom from the cycle of suffering.

muladhara The root chakra (red), located at the base of the spine; governs safety, stability, and self-preservation.

nadis Energetic channels or lines running through the body that move pranic energy.

niyama Personal observances; the second limb of yoga, consisting of five internal practices.

om A sacred sound or syllable used in meditation and chanting.

pingala The main right energetic channel (nadi) in the subtle body, spiraling around the central sushumna nadi.

prakriti Matter or the material world; one of the two fundamental principles in yoga philosophy.

pranayama Breath practice; the fourth limb of yoga, working with the life force through breathing.

pranamaya kosha The breath body; the energetic layer that gives life through both breath and life force.

pratipaksha bhavana Cognitive reappraisal; trying different ways of looking at things by considering alternative explanations.

pratyahara Withdrawal of the senses; the fifth limb of yoga, turning inward and tuning out external distractions.

purusha Pure consciousness or the true self; one of the two fundamental principles in yoga philosophy.

raga Craving or attachment; one of the twin kleshas (with dvesha), the desire for something unavailable.

rajas Energy, excitement, brightness, and spontaneity; one of the three gunas.

sahasrara The crown chakra (violet), located at the top of the head; the destination of rising kundalini energy.

samadhi Bliss or pure awareness; the eighth limb of yoga, the culmination of practice.

samskara Mental impressions or thought patterns; habits that can become ruts when done mindlessly.

santosha Contentment; the second niyama, finding radical happiness despite circumstances.

sattva Balance, light, rightness, and goodness; one of the three gunas.

satya Truth or honesty; the second yama, directing practitioners to be truthful unless it causes harm.

saucha Cleanliness or purity; the first niyama, attending to orderliness and minimizing mess.

savasana Final resting pose in yoga practice; a time of stillness and integration.

sushumna The central energetic channel (nadi) through which kundalini rises from the base of the spine to the crown.

svadhisthana The sacral chakra (orange), located below the belly button; governs emotions, creativity, sensuality, and sexuality.

svadhyaya Self-study and self-knowledge; the fourth niyama, the practice of knowing yourself fully.

tamas Groundedness, lethargy, darkness, and heaviness; one of the three gunas.

tapas Disciplined effort or fiery dedication; the third niyama, the freedom found in discipline.

Upanishads The last portion of the Vedas; mystical texts that distill the ritual ideas of the Vedas into contemplative teachings.

vasana Impressions or tendencies; unconscious compulsions from past experiences that influence present actions.

vayus The five movements or directions of energy in the body.

Vedas Four ancient yogic texts (*Rig Veda*, *Samar Veda*, *Yajur Veda*, and *Atharva Veda*) containing hymns, rituals, and philosophical teachings.

vijnanamaya kosha The intuitive layer; the still, small voice within that holds deep wisdom and gut knowledge.

vishuddha The throat chakra (blue), located at the throat; governs communication and authentic expression.

vritti Fluctuations or modifications of the mind.

yama Ethical restraints; the first limb of yoga, consisting of five external observances.

REFERENCES AND FURTHER STUDY

Now that you've finished this book, you may want to continue your study of yoga philosophy. Fantastic! Here are some other books and films you might look up next. Reading, watching, or listening to media that's not focused specifically on asana is a good way to deepen your practice of yoga off the mat.

Primary Texts

Akers, Brian Dana, trans. *The Hatha Yoga Pradipika*. YogaVidya, 2002.

Desikachar, T. K. V. *The Heart of Yoga*. Inner Traditions, 1999.

Devi, Nischala Joy. *The Secret Power of Yoga*. Harmony Books, 2022.

Easwaran, Eknath, trans. *The Upanishads*. Nilgiri Press, 1987.

Feuerstein, Georg. *The Yoga-Sutra of Patanjali*. Inner Traditions, 1989.

Harvey, Andrew, ed. *The Essential Mystics: Selections from the World's Great Wisdom Traditions*. HarperSanFrancisco, 1996.

Mallinson, James, and Mark Singleton, eds. *Roots of Yoga*. Penguin Classics. Penguin Books, 2017.

Mitchell, Stephen, trans. *Bhagavad Gita: A New Translation*. Harmony Books, 2002.

Odier, Daniel. *Yoga Spandakarika: The Sacred Texts at the Origins of Tantra*. Inner Traditions, 2005.

Roche, Lorin. *The Radiance Sutras: 112 Gateways to the Yoga of Wonder and Delight*. Sounds True, 2014.

Swami Satchidananda, trans. *The Yoga Sutras of Patanjali*. Integral Yoga, 1999.

Secondary Texts

On the History of Yoga

Beres, Derek, and Matthew Remski. *Conspirituality: How New Age Conspiracy Theories Became a Health Threat*. PublicAffairs, 2023.

Carney, Scott. *The Enlightenment Trap: Obsession, Madness and Death on Diamond Mountain*. Foxtopus Ink, 2023.

Patel, Sanjay. *Ramayana: Divine Loophole*. Chronicle Books, 2010.

Roche, Geshe Michael. *How Yoga Works*. Diamond Cutter Press, 2005. (We suggest reading this alongside *The Enlightenment Trap*, listed above, for full context.)

Singleton, Mark. *Yoga Body: The Origins of Modern Posture Practice*. Oxford University Press, 2010.

On Yoga Philosophy

Adele, Deborah. *The Kleshas*. On-Word Bound, 2023.

Adele, Deborah. *The Yamas and Niyamas*. On-Word Bound, 2014.

Balkaran, Raj. *The Stories Behind the Poses: The Indian Mythology That Inspired 50 Yoga Postures*. Leaping Hare Press, 2022.

DiNardo, Kelly, and Amy Pearce-Hayden. *Living the Sutras: A Guide to Yoga Wisdom Beyond the Mat*. Shambhala, 2018.

Jakubowicz, Rina. *The Yoga Mind: 52 Essential Principles of Yoga Philosophy to Deepen Your Practice.* Rockridge Press, 2018.

Johnson, Michelle C. *Illuminating Our True Nature: Yogic Practices for Personal and Collective Healing.* Shambhala, 2024.

Johnson, Michelle C. *Skill in Action: Radicalizing Your Yoga Practice to Create a Just World.* Shambhala, 2021.

Films

Documentaries

This list contains documentaries that shed light on the history and practice of yoga. Please note that there's a long history of abuse of power in yoga. Many new styles arise only to implode in a cloud of scandal. Learning about them will keep your eyes open to the potential pitfalls in studying yoga philosophy with a charismatic teacher.

Breath of Fire, directed by Hayley Pappas and Smiley Stevens (HBO Documentary Films, 2024).

Breath of the Gods: A Journey to the Origins of Modern Yoga, directed by Jan Schmidt-Garre; produced by Marieke Schroeder (PARS Media, 2012).

On Yoga: The Architecture of Peace, directed by Heitor Dhalia (Paranoid Filmes; Michael O'Neill Photography; Urso Filmes, 2017).

Planet Yoga, directed by Carlos Ferrand; produced by InformAction Films and Under The Milky Way (InformAction, 2011).

Wild Wild Country, directed by Chapman Way and Maclain Way (Duplass Brothers Productions, 2018).

Yoga, Inc., directed by John Philp (Bad Dog Tales; Films Transit International, 2007).

Other Films

Enlighten Up! directed by Kate Churchill (Balcony Releasing, 2009). A documentary filmmaker invites a regular guy to attempt to become a yogi.

Kumaré, directed by Vikram Gandhi (Kino Lorber, 2011). A documentary filmmaker poses as a faux guru.

Sita Sings the Blues, directed by Nina Paley (GKIDS, 2008). An animated version of the Ramayana intertwines with the filmmaker's personal life.

Courses/Websites

Raj Balkaran, Indian Wisdom School: www.indianwisdomschool.com.

At Sage's virtual studio, Comfort Zone Yoga, Alexandra leads periodic courses on applying the primary texts of yoga to modern life. Visit www.comfortzoneyoga.com to see the schedule and read more about the teacher trainings we offer.

NOTES

Introduction

1   Georg Feuerstein, *The Yoga Tradition: Its History, Literature, Philosophy and Practice* (Hohm, 2008), 65.

2   Debra Diamond and Molly Emma Aitken, *Yoga: The Art of Transformation* (Smithsonian Institution, 2013), 35.

3   Amy Vaughn, *From the Vedas to Vinyasa* (Opening Lotus Publications, 2016), 22.

4   Crystal Park, Tosca Braun, and Tamar Siegel, "Who Practices Yoga? A Systematic Review of Demographic, Health-Related, and Psychosocial Factors Associated with Yoga Practice," *Journal of Behavioral Medicine* 38, no. 3 (2015): 460–71. https://doi.org/10.1007/s10865-015-9618-5.

5   Svatmarama and Brian Dana Akers, *The Hatha Yoga Pradipika* (YogaVidya.com, 2002), 76.

6   Mark Singleton, *Yoga Body: The Origins of Modern Posture Practice* (Oxford University Press, 2010), 200.

Chapter 5

1   Walt Whitman, "Song of Myself," http://whitmanarchive.org/published/LG/1891/poems/27.

Chapter 6

1 Wendell Berry, *The Mad Farmer Poems* (Counterpoint, 2014), 29–30.

Chapter 7

1 Mihaly Csikszentmihalyi, *Flow: The Psychology of Optimal Experience* (Harper Perennial Modern Classics, 2008).
2 "Yoga Sutra: Sutra 1.19," YogaPradipika, https://www.yogapradipika.com/yoga-sutra-19.

Part II

1 Psychotherapist John Welwood first introduced the term *spiritual bypassing* in his book *Toward a Psychology of Awakening: Buddhism, Psychotherapy, and the Path of Personal and Spiritual Transformation* (Shambhala, 2002).

Chapter 15

1 Walt Whitman, "Song of Myself," http://whitmanarchive.org/published/LG/1891/poems/27.

Chapter 20

1 Hafiz and Daniel Ladinsky, *I Heard God Laughing: Poems of Hope and Joy* (Penguin Publishing Group, 2006), 66.

Chapter 22

1 See Sage's book *The Athlete's Guide to Recovery* (2024) for more.

Chapter 24

1 Georg Feuerstein, *Tantra: The Path of Ecstasy* (Shambhala, 1998).
2 C. W. Leadbeater, *The Chakras: A Monograph* (Quest Books, 1977. Originally published in 1927 by Theosophical Publishing House).
3 Anodea Judith 2004. *Eastern Body, Western Mind: Psychology and the Chakra System as a Path to the Self* (Celestial Arts, 1996), xii.

Chapter 29

1 Stephen Mitchell, trans., *Bhagavad Gita: A New Translation* (Harmony Books, 2002), 55.
2 Mitchell, *Bhagavad Gita*, 147.
3 Mitchell, *Bhagavad Gita*, 148.
4 Victor E. Frankl, *Man's Search for Meaning*, trans. Ilse Lasch. (Beacon Press, 2006), 65.

BIBLIOGRAPHY

Anodea, Judith. *Eastern Body, Western Mind: Psychology and the Chakra System As a Path to the Self.* Ten Speed Press, 2004.

Csikszentmihalyi, Mihaly. *Flow: The Psychology of Optimal Experience.* Harper Perennial Modern Classics, 2008.

Diamond, Debra, and Molly Emma Aitken. *Yoga: The Art of Transformation.* Arthur M. Sackler Gallery, Smithsonian Institution, 2013.

Feuerstein, Georg. *Tantra: The Path of Ecstasy.* Shambhala, 1998.

Feuerstein, Georg. *The Yoga Tradition: Its History, Literature, Philosophy, and Practice.* Hohm Press, 1998; expanded editions, 2001, 2008.

Frankl, Viktor E., Harold S. Kushner, and William J. Winslade. *Man's Search for Meaning.* Beacon Press, 2006.

Hafiz and Daniel Ladinsky. *I Heard God Laughing: Poems of Hope and Joy.* Penguin Publishing Group, 2006.

Katie, Byron. *Loving What Is, Revised Edition: Four Questions That Can Change Your Life; The Revolutionary Process Called "The Work."* Harmony Books, 2021.

Leadbeater, C. W. *The Chakras: A Monograph.* Quest Books, 1977. Originally published in 1927 by Theosophical Publishing House.

Mitchell, Stephen. *Bhagavad Gita: A New Translation.* Harmony Books, 2002.

Park, Crystal L., Tosca Braun, and Tamar Siegel. "Who Practices Yoga? A Systematic Review of Demographic, Health-Related, and Psychosocial Factors Associated with Yoga Practice." *Journal of Behavioral Medicine* 38, no. 3 (January 29, 2015): 460–71. https://doi.org /10.1007/s10865-015-9618-5.

Rountree, Sage. *The Athlete's Guide to Recovery,* Second Edition. Rowman & Littlefield, 2024.

Singleton, Mark. *Yoga Body: The Origins of Modern Posture Practice.* Oxford University Press, 2010.

Svatmarama and Brian Dana Akers. *The Hatha Yoga Pradipika.* YogaVidya.com, 2002.

Vaughn, Amy. *From the Vedas to Vinyasa: An Introduction to the History and Philosophy of Yoga.* Opening Lotus, 2016.

Welwood, John. *Toward a Psychology of Awakening: Buddhism, Psychotherapy, and the Path of Personal and Spiritual Transformation.* Shambhala, 2002.

Whitman, Walt. "Song of Myself." 1891. The Walt Whitman Archive, accessed October 24, 2025. https://whitmanarchive.org/item/ppp.00707_00733.

YogaPradipika. "Yoga Sutra: Sutra 1.19." Accessed September 29, 2025. www.yogapradipika.com/yoga-sutra-19.

INDEX

ABOUT THE AUTHORS

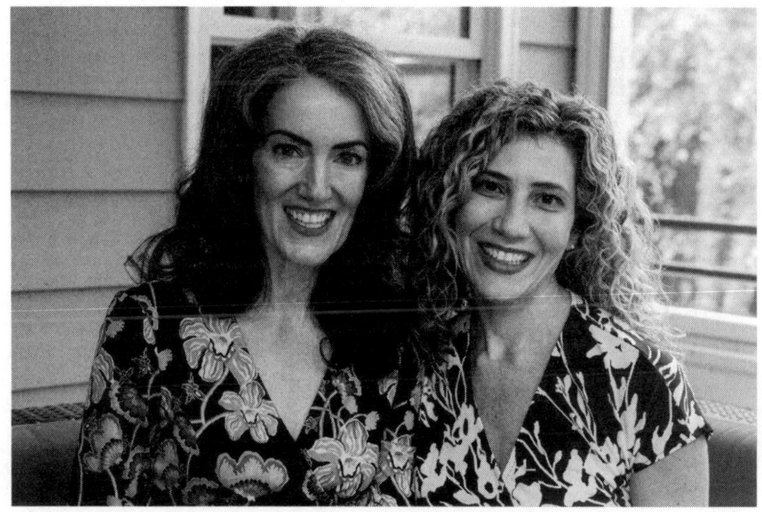

PHOTO BY RADHIKA DESHMUKH-MCDIARMID, RADIAN PHOTOGRAPHY

Sage Rountree holds a PhD in English literature and the highest level of registration with the Yoga Alliance (E-RYT500, YACEP). She directs the Carolina Yoga Company's two-hundred-hour and three-hundred-hour (or five-hundred-hour) teacher trainings. She also offers a robust virtual studio at www.comfortzoneyoga.com, which includes classes, teacher trainings, and retreats. Sage's work gives yoga teachers everything they need to feel confident, relaxed, and helpful in front of the classroom. Her most recent books are *The Art of Yoga Sequencing* (2024) and *The Professional Yoga Teacher's Handbook* (2020). She lives in North Carolina with her husband, Wes.

Alexandra DeSiato is an experienced yoga teacher at the highest level (E-RYT 500). She is also certified in Pilates and has an MA in English literature. Alexandra teaches yoga and has previously led the two-hundred-hour yoga teacher training at Carrboro Yoga Company. Find videos, blog posts, and more at www.alexandradesiato.com. Alexandra has partnered with Sage on three other books: *Lifelong Yoga* (2017), about healthy aging and yoga, and *Teaching Yoga Beyond the Poses* (2019) and *Teaching Yoga Beyond the Poses, Volume 2* (2025), both of which provide inspiration for how to teach the broader concepts of yoga. She is the cocreator of a prenatal- and postpartum-yoga teaching collective, Whole Mama Yoga, and the coauthor of the guidebook *Whole Mama Yoga* (2023). She lives in North Carolina with her husband, daughter, and cat—all of whom support her writing.

ABOUT THE ILLUSTRATOR

Lasha Mutual (https://lashamutual.com) is an artist whose deep commitment to Buddhist theory and practice has suffused her artistic expression, giving rise to a body of work that blends the action of painting with a meditative sense of contemplation and focus. Lasha's intention is to cultivate a generous, peaceful, and clear mind that becomes manifest in her artwork and that can be shared with others. She lives with her husband, her son, and an abundance of pets in a little yellow brick cottage in Stratford, Ontario, Canada.

ABOUT
NORTH ATLANTIC BOOKS

North Atlantic Books (NAB) is an independent, nonprofit publisher committed to a bold exploration of the relationships between mind, body, spirit, and nature. Founded in 1974, NAB aims to nurture a holistic view of the arts, sciences, humanities, and healing. To make a donation or to learn more about our books, authors, events, and newsletter, please visit www.northatlanticbooks.com.